More About Receptors

More About Receptors

Current Reviews in Biomedicine 2

Edited by John W. Lamble

Foreword by A. W. Cuthbert

1982

ELSEVIER BIOMEDICAL PRESS
Amsterdam – New York – Oxford

© 1982 Elsevier Biomedical Press

ISBN: 0-444-80428-5

Published by
Elsevier Biomedical Press BV
P.O. Box 1527
1000 BM Amsterdam
The Netherlands

Sole distributors worldwide except for the U.S.A. and Canada
Elsevier Biomedical Press (Cambridge)
68 Hills Road
Cambridge CB2 1LA
United Kingdom

Sole distributors for the U.S.A. and Canada
Elsevier Science Publishing Company Inc.
52 Vanderbilt Avenue
New York, NY 10017, U.S.A.

PRINTED IN THE UNITED KINGDOM

Foreword

There is nothing, so they say, that succeeds like success. The first collection of papers selected mainly from *Trends in Pharmacological Sciences (TIPS)* and entitled 'Towards Understanding Receptors' which was issued in 1981 proved to be such a successful venture that there is little need to introduce this second collection. The format for 'More About Receptors' is precisely the same as for the former volume, that is, selected, unexpurgated articles from *TIPS* and its sister journals have been arranged in a sensible order and recast in textbook format.

TIPS articles are not reviews in the strict sense and authors are allowed, or even encouraged, to present their own point of view developed from results gathered in their own laboratories. No Tennyson's 'chorus of indolent reviewers' are these writers but hard-headed, practical scientists with a story to tell. Information about receptors is now accumulating at such a rate that pharmacologists need a newspaper to keep abreast of the developments in fields not their own. *TIPS* fills this need and collections of articles, such as this, provide a very convenient format with all the clutter removed. There are, however, some dangers of collecting the articles together between boards, be they hard or soft. It provides an illusion of permanence for what is a collection of 'state of the art' articles. The ephemeral nature of many of the hypotheses will doubtless be revealed in editions of *TIPS* yet to come, and volumes like this one will chronicle the evolutionary paths of modern pharmacology.

Few pharmacologists will find nothing to interest them in this collection, while most who are concerned with the molecular aspects of receptors will wish to keep the volume close by. The succinct style of the articles, not overburdened with references, make it a very handy book for both graduate and undergraduate students, and keen-eyed examiners will have noticed that student essays can have a more than superficial resemblance to *TIPS* articles.

Two articles on membrane receptors and hormone action by Hollenberg, the first dealing with structure and regulation and the second with function, provide a convenient opening scenario. Indeed, so wide is the coverage in these chapters that they could have served as an appropriate foreword to the whole collection. In an article I wrote in the inaugural issue of *TIPS*[1] I suggested that progress in understanding receptors had been hindered by the ease with which drug responses can be recorded using simple physiological systems, leading to an excessive concern with 'autonomic' receptors. These seemingly straightforward measurements were, of course, very far removed from the actual interactions between drug and receptor. Hollenberg's articles show just how far progress has been made and it is refreshing that receptors for, say, epidermal growth factor are mentioned alongside nicotinic receptors, even though the 'response' to activation of the former is complex and ill-understood. What is important to Hollenberg is the receptor, what it is made of, how it works and is regulated. One cannot help but feel hopeful that general principles about receptor mechanisms will eventually emerge from the mass of information now being collected. One principle that is fast becoming established as a general mechanism of receptors relates to their dynamic nature, a theme pursued in some detail in a later contribution by Perkins. Receptor properties and membrane densities are now known to change in response to a variety of perturbations with, of course, dramatic consequences for the relationship between drug concentration and response. The need to make measurements as close as possible to the receptor events is ever pressing; ligand binding and patch clamping are techniques which have already contributed much in this respect. At the end of the second article by Hollenberg some of the questions for future research are posed. The techniques that will be required are to some extent obvious and pharmacologists must do what they always have done, that is, borrow them from other disciplines if they are appropriate.

One way in which receptor occupation can be translated into a cellular response is via adenylate cyclase, which properly continues to occupy a front-line position in receptor research. Several papers on this topic are included here. Levitzki describes the intricacies of the interactions between receptor, GTP binding protein and the catalytic subunit of adenylate cyclase. Another paper, by Porzig, points to the importance of cellular studies as well as the 'grind and bind' approach, highlighting important differences which have arisen from experiments in the β-receptor-adenylate cyclase system of whole cells and homogenates. 'Anti-idiotype' antibodies (anti-antihormone antibodies) have been used by the immunology group of CNRS in Paris to look at the β-receptor-adenylate cyclase complex. This is a novel approach which has also been applied to the insulin receptor and it will be interesting to see how far this technique can be applied to other systems. In general, pharmacologists have been rather slow to exploit immunological techniques for receptor problems. Development and use of monoclonal antibodies and anti-antihormone antibodies for the demonstration, localization and isolation of membrane receptors are obvious ways forward. An article from *Immunology Today*, a sister publication to *TIPS*, is included in this collection for those who may wish to become a little more familiar with these approaches.

The role of cAMP in the nervous system and in synaptic transmission is considered in two other contributions. It is pointed out that there are many steps in the process between cAMP generation and the pharmacological response, involving, for example, cAMP-dependent protein kinases or protein phosphatases, which have yet to be targets for drug action. Recent reports on the actions of the diterpene forskolin, apparently a direct activator of the catalytic subunit of adenylate cyclase[2], are perhaps an indication that other steps in the cascade, beyond the initial recognition events, are pharmacologically amenable.

It is intriguing that in the adrenoceptor area the variety of drugs available and their specificity seems inversely related to the period of study. Only one paper is included on α-receptors, by Exton. He concludes that the presynaptic α_2-receptors are operated by unknown molecular mechanisms, post-synaptic α_2-receptors inhibit adenylate cyclase by uncertain mechanisms while post-synaptic α_1-receptors may operate through activating calcium gates or the ubiquitous phosphatidylinositol (PI) mechanism. On the other hand, for the dopamine receptor, which is quite the baby of the adrenoceptor family, one is spoilt for choice. It is proving difficult to classify dopamine receptors, or even it seems, to decide a basis for classification. Three papers on this topic are included in this volume, and while there is a deal of common ground between them there are subtle differences. It is right that the reader should be exposed to the three points of view and, furthermore, all the three articles by Cools, by Beart and by Offermeier and van Rooyen should be consumed at one reading.

Very low concentrations of apomorphine inhibit dopamine synthesis in the striatum and limbic system. This paradoxical effect has been linked to the activation of dopamine (presynaptic) autoreceptors. Nilsson and Carlsson describe in their article the actions of a new compound, 3PPP, which is apparently highly specific for dopamine autoreceptors and which fails to have post-synaptic actions at near lethal doses. The possibility of obtaining selective antipsychotic actions without troublesome extrapyramidal side effects is exciting.

No collection of articles on membrane receptors would be complete without something about GABA receptors. The relation between benzodiazepine binding sites and GABA receptors is well known and in his article Möhler considers whether or not there are endogenous ligands for the binding sites for benzodiazepines. Barbiturate drugs also affect the interaction of GABA with its receptors and Johnston and Willow propose that the barbiturate receptor may be a lipid, in their article on barbiturate receptors.

The ways in which muscarinic acetylcholine receptors are coupled to their final effector process is unclear. It has, of course, been known for 20 years or so that activation of muscarinic receptors in different situations can lead to very different biophysical events, for example, an increase in potassium ion permeability leads to hyperpolarization in the heart while in smooth muscle a depolarization results from an increase in permeability to sodium and/or calcium ions. Also, the response to muscarinic receptor activation is relatively slow suggesting that, in some instances at least, coupling via metabolic processes is required. This theme is pursued by Hartzell in his paper on the physiological consequences of muscarinic receptor activation.

It is to be remembered that the first detailed ligand binding study was made on the muscarinic receptor using ^{14}C-labelled atropine[3]. A variety of reversible ligands with affinities greater than those of atropine are now available as well as rather specific irreversible compounds such as the benzilylcholine mustards. A view of the muscarinic receptor gained from ligand binding studies is given in a paper by Sokolovsky and Bartfai, one of two papers in this volume taken from *Trends in Biochemical Sciences (TIBS)*.

No matter where they are located, nicotinic receptors when activated cause a rapidly developing, short lasting increase in membrane permeability with very little ion selectivity. It seems likely, therefore, that the recognition site of the nicotinic receptor is closely associated with a membrane ionophore. As a consequence it is feasible to examine both binding studies and simultaneous ion fluxes by use of a suitable membrane vesicle preparation. This is precisely what Taylor and Sine have done in order to study the relation between occupancy and activation of the permeability mechanism.

Non-imidazole histamine H_2-antagonists are the subject of the only paper on histamine receptors in this volume.

Ever since it was found that adenosine could modify adenylate cyclase activity the possibility of the existence of physiologically relevant adenosine receptors has been explored. What has been learned from direct binding studies using non-metabolizable ligands is reviewed by Schwabe.

Although no papers on the insulin receptor were included in 'Towards Understanding Receptors', results with this receptor continue to raise intriguing questions such as, 'why is the insulin receptor complex internalized?', 'is internalization essential for coupling the membrane event with the effector system?' and 'is the insulin receptor complex responsible for directing the insertion of glucose transporting activity from the Golgi to membrane and, if so, what are the second messengers?' The earlier omission has been rectified by including a paper on insulin action and one on structural features of the receptor, the second of these coming from *TIBS*.

The involvement of membrane lipids in drug action is not a new concept but their precise role is yet to be formulated. A paper by Cockcroft further explores the Michell hypothesis that breakdown of PI as a result of receptor activation is responsible for calcium gating. One cannot help but feel a sense of *déjà vu* when reading the literature on PI breakdown and I had cause to reread what I had written on this topic in a review in 1967[4]. The Hokins had done much to establish the mechanism of drug-mediated PI turnover in the mid-1950s and had suggested that it might be involved in sodium ion translocation. Indeed it was a disappointment to find that oxytocin, which stimulates sodium transport in toad bladder, does not cause ^{32}P incorporation into phospholipids. On the other hand, acetylcholine did stimulate ^{32}P incorporation but was not shown to stimulate sodium transport[5]. Now it is recognized that the oxytocin effect is mediated by cyclic AMP, and no other receptor known to stimulate adenylate cyclase has been shown to stimulate PI turnover. Furthermore, high-resistance sodium transporting epithelia have now been shown to respond to acetylcholine under appropriate circumstances[6]. Thus some of the data, which led earlier investigators to abandon the idea that PI turnover was associated with sodium ion translocation, can now be seen to fit well the criteria of the Michell hypothesis. Nevertheless the question still remains one of cause or effect. Cockcroft points out that ATP-induced histamine secretion from mast cells is calcium dependent but, in the absence of calcium, the PI response does not occur. In this instance it would seem that the PI response is an effect, rather than the cause of the calcium influx! More recent studies from Michell's laboratories have concentrated on the reactions of triphosphoinositides with impressive calcium chelating activity. Doubtless a later collection of papers from *TIPS* will have a contribution on this topic.

Histamine release from mast cells is also the subject of the paper by Axelrod and Hirata. Concanavalin A stimulation of mast cells leads to the progressive methylation of phosphatidylethanolamine to phosphatidylcholine, an event which precedes both Ca^{2+} influx and histamine release. Inhibitors of the methyltransferases involved in the methylation reactions also inhibit Ca^{2+} influx and release of histamine. These authors have developed a particularly elegant way of demonstrating the importance of the transferase reactions without the use of drugs. Rat basophilic leukaemia cell lines were isolated which were deficient in either methyltransferase I or methyltransferase II activity and unable to release histamine with the usual stimuli. After the cells were fused to form a hybrid, histamine releasing capacity was restored. A full account of this approach has now appeared[7].

The last paper in this volume presents an unusual riddle. Using the guinea-pig papillary muscle Ebner has demonstrated a propranolol resistant inotropic effect which is blocked by hydrocortisone. Arguing from the known effects of these drugs the author is forced to conclude that part of the inotropic effect comes from activation of intracellular receptors. Receptors, like other membrane macromolecules, must be synthesized by the cell and inserted into the membrane after passing through the usual processing arrangements. The possibility that receptors can be activated before insertion in the cell membrane and, more mysteriously, be coupled to an effector process does not fit within the present framework of thinking about adrenoceptors. Clearly there is a challenge here for future authors of *TIPS* articles to pursue these interesting findings.

It has been a pleasure for me to reread these articles for inclusion in this volume. G. Alan Robison wrote in the foreword to the first volume, 'many authors have let their interest and exitement show through'; this is no less true of this collection. It is fun to read and, in my view, a true picture of the 'state of the art'.

A. W. CUTHBERT
Cambridge

References

1 Cuthbert, A. W. (1979) *Trends Pharmacol. Sci., Inaugural issue*, 1, 1–3
2 Seamon, K. and Daly, J. W. (1981) *J. Biol. Chem.* 10, 9799–9801
3 Paton, W. D. M. and Rang, H. P. (1965) *Proc. Roy. Soc. B* 163, 1–44
4 Cuthbert, A. W. (1967) *Pharmacol. Rev.* 19, 59–106
5 Hestrin-Lerner, S. and Hokin, L. E. (1964) *Amer. J. Physiol.* 206, 136–142
6 Cuthbert, A. W. and Wilson, S. A. (1981) *J. Memb. Biol.* 59, 65–75
7 McGivney, A., Crews, F. T., Hirata, F., Axelrod, J. and Siraganian, R. P. (1981) *Proc. Natl Acad. Sci. U.S.A.* 78, 6176–6180

Preface

This second volume of papers about receptors, selected from Elsevier magazines, appears less than 12 months after the first. Growth of knowledge in this area is tremendous and for this reason alone a second book would be justified. However, it should also be stressed that *More About Receptors* and *Towards Understanding Receptors* are largely complementary, and many themes appear in this volume which were not covered before.

Although most papers reproduced here have been taken from *Trends in Pharmacological Sciences*, two come from *Trends in Biochemical Sciences* and one comes from *Immunology Today*. This emphasizes that it is topics like receptor studies, in which various disciplines mingle and cross-fertilize each other with paradigms and techniques, which represent the most dynamic growth areas of science. One inhibitor of such interactions is the specialized jargon which permeates so much scientific literature. It is thus a pleasure to report the efforts of authors whose papers are published here, to minimize this feature and thus provide much enjoyable reading.

I am glad, also, to express my deep gratitude to Professor A. W. Cuthbert for his advice during the assembly of the book and for his contribution of an excellent foreword.

JOHN W. LAMBLE

Contents

Foreword, *A. W. Cuthbert*	v
Editor's Preface	x
Membrane receptors and hormone action I: new trends related to receptor structure and receptor regulation, *Morley D. Hollenberg*	1
Membrane receptors and hormone action II: new perspectives for receptor-modulated cell function, *Morley D. Hollenberg*	7
Activation and inhibition of adenylate cyclase by hormones: mechanistic aspects, *Alexander Levitzki*	14
Are there differences in the β-receptor-adenylate cyclase systems of fragmented membranes and living cells?, *Hartmut Porzig*	25
Biochemical and immunochemical analysis of β-adrenergic receptor adenylate cyclase complexes, *A. Donny Strosberg, P. O. Couraud, O. Durieu-Trautmann and C. Delavier-Klutchko*	32
Immunological studies of hormone receptors: a two-way approach, *A. Donny Strosberg, P.-Olivier Couraud and Alain Schreiber*	40
Catecholamine-induced modification of the functional state of β-adrenergic receptors, *John P. Perkins*	48
Proving a role for cyclic AMP in synaptic transmission, *Clark A. Briggs and Donald A. McAfee*	54
Cyclic nucleotides and the nervous system, *Tamas Bartfai*	61
Molecular mechanisms involved in α-adrenergic responses, *John H. Exton*	66
The puzzling 'cascade' of multiple receptors for dopamine: an appraisal of the current situation, *A. R. Cools*	76
Multiple dopamine receptors – new vistas, *Philip M. Beart*	87
Is it possible to integrate dopamine receptor terminology?, *Johan Offermeier and Johlene M. van Rooyen*	93
Dopamine-receptor agonist with apparent selectivity for autoreceptors: a new principle for antipsychotic action?, *J. Lars G. Nilsson and Arvid Carlsson*	98
Benzodiazepine receptors: are there endogenous ligands in the brain?, *H. Möhler*	105
GABA and barbiturate receptors, *Graham A. R. Johnston and Max Willow*	111
Physiological consequences of muscarinic receptor activation, *H. Criss Hartzell*	115
Biochemical studies on muscarinic receptors, *Mordechai Sokolovsky and Tamas Bartfai*	119
Ligand occupation and the functional states of the nicotinic-cholinergic receptor, *Palmer Taylor and Steven M. Sine*	125

Recent developments in histamine H_2-antagonists, *R. T. Brittain, D. Jack and B. J. Price* — 134

Direct binding studies of adenosine receptors, *Ulrich Schwabe* — 140

The controversial problem of insulin action, *Otto Walaas and Robert S. Horn* — 148

The insulin receptor: structural features, *Michael P. Czech, Joan Massague and Paul F. Pilch* — 154

Does phosphatidylinositol breakdown control the Ca^{2+}-gating mechanism?, *S. Cockcroft* — 162

Phospholipid methylation and the receptor-induced release of histamine from cells, *Julius Axelrod and Fusao Hirata* — 167

Putatively intracellular adrenoceptors contribute to the positive inotropic effect of noradrenaline, *F. Ebner* — 172 # Membrane receptors and hormone action I: new trends related to receptor structure and receptor regulation

Morley D. Hollenberg

Department of Pharmacology and Therapeutics, Faculty of Medicine, University of Calgary, Calgary, Alberta Canada, T2N 1N4.

Introduction

Along with other rapidly developing areas of cell biology, the study of receptor*-related mechanisms that lead to cell activation is undergoing a veritable metamorphosis. Great strides have been made since the development of the receptor concept at the turn of the century (from 'fiction, to fact', as detailed elsewhere[1,2]), to the point where biochemical details about several of the protein oligomers responsible for ligand recognition are becoming available; and where for certain systems, the individual membrane-localized reactions that occur subsequent to ligand binding are being elucidated. It would be impossible for a single review to document with justice all of the very many exciting studies that are continually appearing to describe the molecular characteristics of receptors for an ever widening number of ligands; almost without exception, the study of each receptor yields some surprises and brings to light more challenges. Rather, an attempt will be made to use selected examples of studies that illustrate the kind of progress that has been made over the past few years and that point to new areas of potential development. In this first article, the focus will be on receptor structure and receptor regulation; a subsequent article will deal with receptor-modulated cell function. For reasons of economy, attention will be focused on those receptors that are localized in the plasma membrane.

The status quo

Before proceeding, it is useful to give a synopsis of the present picture of membrane receptor function. Methods are well in hand for receptor identification, both by pharmacological and biochemical (primarily ligand binding) methods[3]. To date, most of the recognition molecules appear to be rather large oligomeric protein† species, that in detergent solution exhibit mol. wts in the 100,000–300,000 range; the size of the individual recognition subunits varies from about 40,000 (acetylcholine receptor) to about 180,000 (receptor for epidermal growth factor-urogastrone). The receptors appear to be in a dynamic rather

---

* The term receptor is used here in a restricted sense to denote a molecule that exhibits the dual function of ligand recognition and cell activation.

† Note however the ability of small non-protein molecules, e.g. gangliosides, to function as binding substituents or receptors for certain toxins and hormones[4].

than a static state, both in terms of the turnover of these membrane-localized substituents (*de novo* synthesis, insertion, internalization and 'processing') and in terms of the mobility of certain receptors within the plane of the plasma membrane. The mobility of certain receptors may be relatively restricted (e.g. those, like the acetylcholine receptor that modulate a localized ion channel), whereas other receptors (e.g. those that modulate adenylate cyclase) appear to have comparatively unrestricted mobility, so as to permit a variety of interactions with other membrane-localized substituents. There are a number of theories of receptor function (reviewed in some depth elsewhere[1-3,5]) that take into account both receptor mobility and the multipoint/allosteric nature of ligand binding. In essence, the functions of receptors like other oligomeric proteins can be understood in terms of regulatory mechanisms that have been observed to operate in a variety of multi-enzyme systems; the challenge lies in finding the appropriate enzymatic paradigm that best matches the idiosyncracies of a particular receptor system. This is not to say that the documentation of new receptor mechanisms will not require novel insight, but rather that the recognized enzyme-like nature of receptor interactions provides a rich point of departure for those facile with complex enzymatic mechanisms. In brief, many membrane receptors can be viewed as complex, mobile enzyme-like oligomers that function in a restricted membrane environment.

While the above synopsis may be an oversimplification of an 'obvious' state of affairs, it is fair to say that it has taken about 80 years to arrive at the point where this explicit statement can be made with any confidence (notwithstanding the recognized shortcomings of our present understanding). Where, then, does one go from here? On a comprehensive 'wish list', one would aim for more in-depth studies of several selected receptor systems. More information is needed about the molecular structure of receptors (sequence, common regions in different receptors, overall conformation), about functions that govern receptor regulation (both at the genetic and epigenetic level) about the kind of information stored in the receptor *per se*, about the detailed series of protein–protein interactions that lead from ligand recognition to a specific cellular response, and about the relationship of receptor structure and function to the pathogenesis of certain disease states. The lessons learned about hormone receptor structure and function may well apply to other membrane constituents (antibodies, cell–cell recognition sites) that modulate cellular function.

Receptor structure

Except for the nicotinic receptor for acetycholine, the amounts of receptor material available for study usually preclude the use of direct chemical analysis (amino acid analysis, sequence, etc.). Nonetheless, a great deal of information has been obtained with the use of the specific high affinity ligands as receptor 'markers', along with photoaffinity and affinity-crosslinking labeling methods, enzymatic probe techniques and lectin-probe methods. Thus, data obtained for receptors for polypeptides such as insulin or epidermal growth factor-urogastrone (EGF-URO) indicate that the receptors are glycoproteins that are only partially embedded in the membrane lipid environment. It is interesting to note that important functional information resides both in the protein and non-protein constituents of receptors. It is now evident, for instance, that the oligosaccharide portion of receptors may play a role both in the ligand recognition function (e.g. removal of sialic acid augments the binding of EGF-URO to its receptor) and in the signal-transduction process (e.g. neuraminidase abrogates insulin action in adipocytes without affecting insulin binding). A contribution of other non-protein moieties (possibly, tightly receptor-associated via non-covalent mechanisms) to ligand recognition can be seen in the likely participation of gangliosides in the binding and action of agents such as thyroid stimulating hormone and interferon[4].

In terms of protein structure, new data for the insulin receptor indicate that two or more polypeptide chains appear to be involved in ligand recognition (data summarized in several communications in Ref. 6). On the one hand, photolabeling and affinity crosslinking methods have been used in the laboratories of M. Czech, S. Jacobs, M. Wisher, C. C. Yip and others[6], to identify a ligand recognition species (alpha-chain) that upon electrophoresis under reducing conditions exhibits a mol. wt of about 135,000; electrophoresis under non-reducing conditions indicates that the labeled constituent behaves as a species with a mol. wt somewhat above 300,000. Crosslinking experiments, using disuccinimidyl suberate[6] indicate that, upon binding to the receptor, insulin is also in proximity to a second polypeptide (beta-chain) that, under reducing conditions, has a mol. wt of about 90,000. Limited reduction of the insulin-labeled receptor yields a species with a mol. wt in the 200,000 range. On the other hand, these data obtained by ligand-crosslinking methods are complemented by the detection of similar protein constituents, upon analysis of insulin receptor that has been highly purified by affinity-chromatographic methods[6]. Taken together, the data indicate an oligomeric structure of the insulin receptor, with a two-chain ligand recognition species $(\alpha\beta)$ that may exist in the membrane as a disulfide-linked multimer $(\alpha\beta)_2$. For insulin, the ligand recognition event may turn out to be a very complicated process, including not only the participation of a number of polypeptide chains comprising the receptor recognition oligomer *per se*, but also including input from other 'non-recognition' or 'non-receptor' glycoprotein moieties with which the receptor oligomer can interact.

Even more detailed information about receptor structure–function relationships can be anticipated from studies with the nicotinic-cholinergic receptor[7], for which substantial amounts of material can be obtained from *Torpedo* and *electroplax* species. In detergent solutions, the receptor behaves as a species with an apparent mol. wt of about 250,000; the entire oligomeric structure $(\alpha_2\beta\gamma\delta)$ comprises two recognition subunits (α, mol. wt about 40,000) and an oligomer $(\beta\gamma\delta)$ (possibly the ion channel) composed of three distinct, but chemically-related[8] substituents with mol. wts of about 48,000 (β), 58,000 (γ) and 64,000 (δ)[7]. As the detailed structures of the ligand recognition components and the ion channel species become available, it should be possible to improve our understanding of the complex interactions of agonists, partial agonists, antagonists and ion-channel-specific agents that modulate the ion transport function of this complex oligomeric receptor.

Receptor regulation

It is now apparent, as reviewed in some detail elsewhere[2], that cell surface receptors for a variety of agents can be modulated at one of several levels. In cells like quiescent lymphocytes, cell activation (antibody, plant lectin) can lead to the *de novo* appearance of receptors, such as the one for insulin. Further, the appearance of specific receptors, and the coupling of receptors to effector systems (e.g. adenylate cyclase, cation transport systems) can be observed to be developmentally related. For instance, in mouse embryos, receptors for epidermal growth factor increase during gestation, with a pronounced effect evident in a target tissue such as the maxilla[9]. Similarly, for β-nerve growth factor in the chick, receptor content and β-nerve growth factor responsiveness vary with development. In maturing rat erythrocytes, catecholamine responsiveness (adenylate cyclase) decreases markedly, without concomitant changes in the erythrocyte receptor content. Presumably in many instances of this kind related to development, changes in receptor content and function will be found to be hormonally regulated at the genetic level (e.g. steroid hormones can control the receptors for peptide hormones). Apart from changes related to a developmental process, changes in the receptor for one hormone can be regulated by a second hormone. This kind of regulation may be termed 'heterospecific' receptor regulation, in which the process is distinct from the control of receptor internalization (see below)[10]. Heterospecific hormone receptor regulation represents an important control point for a variety of biological processes and, therefore, represents a fascinating area for future research. As nucleic acid probes become available for receptor-related research, it may be possible to study this aspect of the control of receptor biosynthesis at the genetic level. Such studies will complement the methods already available for monitoring receptor turnover (heavy isotope methods) and membrane insertion (conventional ligand binding methods). In brief, given the availability of antireceptor antibodies (see below) and given the recent advances in molecular biology, it would appear that a new threshold of sophistication in the analysis of receptor regulation may be at hand.

Evidence is now emerging for a kind of heterospecific receptor regulation that is distinct from control at the genetic level. The site of this control appears to be localized within the plasma membrane. For instance, work from the laboratories of I. B. Weinstein, G. J. Todaro, E. Rozengurt and others (summarized in Ref. 11) indicates that the tumor promoter, 12-0-tetradecanoylphorbol-13-acetate (TPA), interacting with its own distinct membrane receptor, causes a rapid (tens of minutes) time- and temperature-dependent selective reduction of cell receptors for EGF-URO. Evidence has also been obtained for a heterospecific regulatory interaction (up- and down-regulation) between the receptors for EGF-URO, platelet-derived growth factor and fibroblast growth factor[12]. In contrast, carbachol, acting via a muscarinic receptor in rat cardiac tissue can increase the affinity of the α_1-adrenoceptor for the α-adrenergic antagonist ligand WB4101 [2-N(2,6 dimethoxyphenoxyethyl) aminomethyl-1,4-benzodioxane][13]; the muscarinic agonist partially reverses the decrease in α_1-receptor ligand affinity caused by the guanine nucleotide analogue, guanyl-5'-imidodiphosphate (GMP-P(NH)P). Another intriguing example of this kind can be seen in the insulin-mediated augmentation of the binding of the insulin-like growth factors, multiplication stimulating activity (MSA) and basic-somatomedin by rat adipocytes[14,15]. For MSA, the increase in receptor binding caused by insulin receptor occupation is due to an increase in MSA ligand affinity; the effect is time- and temperature-dependent and requires an intact cell. A final striking example of membrane-localized heterospecific receptor regulation is evident in the complex reciprocal relationship between the binding of gamma-aminobutyric acid (GABA) and the benzodiazepines in isolated membrane preparations (summarized in Refs 16–18). The binding data are consistent with previously obtained electrophysiological evidence indicating that diazepam augments GABA-mediated inhibitory effects on neurons. The increase in [³H]GABA binding caused by diazepam, and the augmentation of [³H]methyl-diazepam binding in the presence of GABA can be observed within minutes in isolated membrane preparations. The effect of diazepam on GABA binding has been attributed to its ability to complex with a separate non-receptor endogenous membrane-associated thermostable component (GABA modulin; mol. wt about 15,000) that reduces the GABA receptor's affinity for GABA; the mechanism whereby GABA affects diazepam binding is not known. It is of interest that, upon solubilization of GABA receptor-containing membranes, both the GABA-binding and diazepam binding activities appear to be associated during purification. It is thus possible that in the intact cell, the various components responsible for the complex GABA/diazepam heterospecific reciprocal receptor regulatory process may exist as a large oligomeric structure. The above examples illustrate a relatively recently discovered type of heterospecific receptor regulation. It will be of great interest in future work to look for similar regulatory processes in other receptor systems.

In addition to heterospecific receptor regulation, it is well recognized that certain hormones can modulate the cell content of their own receptors (this can be termed 'homospecific' up- or down-regulation). For instance, brief (tens of minutes) exposure of cells to epidermal growth factor leads to a marked reduction in cellular binding of EGF-URO; the return of cellular binding activity occurs slowly (tens of hours). In contrast, prolactin appears to cause an up-regulation of its own receptors. In the case of EGF-URO, receptor down-regulation can be clearly correlated with receptor occupation. The sequence of events appears to comprise: receptor binding, lateral mobility of receptors to sites of internalization (? coated pits), endocytosis (possibly involving membrane transglutaminase) and lysosomal fusion of internalized receptor-containing vesicles. In the course of internalization, the receptor is subject to proteolysis (or 'processing'); the significance of the internalization process in terms of cell activation is uncertain. Comparatively little is known about the control of the internalization/receptor degradation process. However, it appears that several hormone receptors may be internalized via a similar, receptor-triggered process[10]. Since receptors for insulin, EGF-URO and α-2-macroglobulin can be observed to co-migrate to the same membrane site prior to internalization, one can reasonably predict that on distinct receptor oligomers, common polypeptide regions will be found that participate in the endocytotic process.

There are also non-hormonal factors that modulate cellular receptor function and content. For instance, viral transforming agents or chemicals such as sodium butyrate can cause both qualitative as well as quantitative alterations in cell receptors. Further, the saturation density of cultured cells can modulate receptor content either in a positive or negative direction; the mechanism whereby cell–cell contact alters receptor number will be a fruitful subject for future study. Most interestingly, it now appears that the extracellular matrix upon which cells sit may govern not only cell receptor content, but also may determine the cellular response upon receptor occupation[19,20]. The control of receptor function by matrix constituents (glycosaminoglycans, fibronectin, collagens) provides an intriguing regulatory process, whereby one hormone, acting at its receptor to stimulate cell matrix production can, via an indirect process, modulate the action of a second hormone acting at a distinct receptor site.

From the above discussion, it is evident that the numbers and characteristics of cell surface receptors can be affected by a large number of factors related both to intracellular events (rates of receptor synthesis and turnover, cell cycle, cell differentiation) and to a variety of extracellular stimuli caused by hormones and other agents. These stimuli may be caused either by hormone receptor occupation (homospecific or heterospecific regulation) or by other non-hormonal cellular effectors (chemical, viruses, extracellular matrix, cell–cell contact).

From the above discussion it is evident that, over a relatively short time period, work on receptors has progressed far beyond the comparatively simple 'grind and bind' experiments of the early 1970s. The affinity labeling methods are now being applied in a number of receptor systems; one can thus predict that very interesting information (e.g. molecular weight; oligomeric composition) about the recognition molecules of a variety of hormone receptors will soon appear. Further, one may anticipate that new insights related to receptor modulation may provide a basis for understanding certain drug–drug interactions at a level that hitherto was not possible.

A question unanswered by this article is: how do receptor structures and receptor dynamics relate to cell activation? A subsequent article will attempt to deal with some aspects of this question.

Reading list

1 Ariëns, E. J. (1979) *Trends Pharmacol. Sci.* 1, 11–15
2 Hollenberg, M. D. (1979) *Pharmacol. Rev.* 30, 393–410
3 Cuatrecasas, P. and Hollenberg, M. D. (1976) *Adv. Protein Chem.* 30, 251–451
4 Kohn, L. D. (1978) in *Cell Receptor Disorders* (Melnechuk, T., ed.), pp. 28–38, Western Behavioural Sciences Inst., La Jolla, CA
5 O'Brien, R. D. (ed) (1979) *The Receptors, a Comprehensive Treatise*, Vol. 1, General Principles and Procedures, Plenum Publishing Corp., New York
6 Andreani, D. and DePirro, R. (eds) (1981) *Current Views on Insulin Receptors*, Proc. 1st int. Symp. Insulin Receptors, Rome, Sept. 1980, Academic Press, New York (in press)
7 Karlin, A. (1980) in *The Cell Surface and Neuronal Function* (Cotman, C. W., Poste, G. and Nicolson, G. L., eds), pp. 191–260, Elsevier/North-Holland Biomedical Press
8 Raftery, M. A., Hunkapiller, M. W., Strader, C. D. and Hood, L. E. (1980) *Science* 208, 1454–1456
9 Nexø, E., Hollenberg, M. D., Figueroa, A. and Pratt, R. M. (1980) *Proc. Natl Acad. Sci. U.S.A.* 77, 2782–2785
10 Pastan, I. and Willingham, M. C. (1981) *Annu. Rev. Physiol.* 43, 239–250
11 Hollenberg, M. D., Nexø, E., Berhanu, P. and Hock, R. A. (1981) in *Receptor-Mediated Binding and Internalization of Toxins and Hormones*, (Middlebrook, J. L. and Kohn, L. D., eds), pp. 181–195, Academic Press, New York
12 Wrann, M., Fox, C. F. and Ross, R. (1980) *Science* 210, 1363–1365
13 Yamada, S., Yamamura, H. I. and Roeske, W. R. (1980) *Eur. J. Pharmacol.* 63, 239–241
14 Bhaumick, B., Goren, H. J. and Bala, R. M. (1981) *Horm. Metab. Res.* (in press)
15 King, G. L., Kahn, C. R. and Rechler, M. M. (1980) *Abstracts, 62nd Meeting, Endocrine Soc.*, Washington, DC, June 1980, p. 145
16 Müller, W. E. (1981) *Pharmacology* 22, 153–161
17 Braestrup, C. and Nielsen, M. (1980) *Drug Res.* 30, 852–857
18 Guidotti, A., Baraldi, M. and Costa, E. (1979) *Pharmacology* 19, 267–277
19 Skehan, P. and Friedman, S. J. (1975) *Exp. Cell Res.* 92, 350–360
20 Gospodarowicz, D., Delgado, D. and Vlodavsky, I. (1980) *Proc. Natl. Acad. Sci. U.S.A.* 77, 4094–4098

Membrane receptors and hormone action II: new perspectives for receptor-modulated cell function

Morley D. Hollenberg

Department of Pharmacology and Therapeutics, Faculty of Medicine, University of Calgary, Calgary, Alberta T2N 1N4, Canada

Introduction

In my previous article[1], attention was focussed on recently-described aspects of receptor structure and on the regulation of the density of cell-surface receptors for polypeptide hormones. A major related area of interest concerns the coupling mechanisms, whereby receptor occupation is translated into a cellular response. Although such coupling reactions may be as diverse as the ligand modulators themselves, it is very possible that there may be membrane-localized processes in common that relate to the activation of the adenylate cyclase system, to antigen-directed cell activation and to the mechanisms whereby hormones like insulin alter cell metabolism.

This article will address some of the interesting new observations that have been made concerning receptor-modulated cell function. It is hoped that progress in this area may have a direct bearing on our understanding of a variety of pathological states that may stem from some aspect of receptor dysfunction.

Receptor-modulated adenylate cyclase

One of the most exciting, rapidly developing areas of receptor research deals with mechanisms whereby a ligand–receptor interaction modulates cellular adenylate cyclase. It was mainly the analysis of the hormone-specific stimulation of adenylate cyclase by several different hormones in the same cell system that led a number of investigators to postulate a 'floating' or 'mobile receptor' model of hormone action (summarized in Refs 2 and 3). The evidence for the independent nature of the hormone recognition molecule, the enzyme catalytic subunit and the 'coupling subunit' (the so-called G-G/F or N-subunit of the cyclase system), which three species form the functional cyclase unit, has been adequately summarized elsewhere[3,4]. The mobility of the receptors, suggested upon theoretical grounds, has been elegantly substantiated for the cyclase system via receptor (glucagon, β-adrenergic) transfer experiments, using cell and membrane fusion methods to reconstitute hormone-modulated cyclase systems from membrane or cell substituents that lack either the hormone receptor or the active cyclase. Whether or not the receptor-induced modulation is via a direct physical interaction with the GTP regulatory subunit remains an open question.

The implications of these models and observations related to the cyclase system are far-ranging. For instance, since different hormone receptors can interact with the same cyclase system, one can predict with some confidence that there must be homologous structural regions in the different cyclase-related receptors. Further, one may postulate that hormones of the 'non-cyclase' class (e.g. insulin) which are known to reduce the cellular levels of cyclic AMP, via an inhibition of the cyclase, have receptors that may in some way interact with the regulatory subunit of the cyclase system[4,5]. In addition, since a receptor from one species (avian erythrocytes) can, after membrane fusion, modulate the cyclase of a second species (mammalian adrenal cell), one can predict that homologous polypeptide sequences will also be present in the cyclase components of different species. Thus, just as there is conservation of important structural regions of polypeptide hormones, one can predict there may also be an evolutionary conservation of the receptor/effector structures that mediate hormone action. A future trend in the study of the cyclase system, therefore, would appear to focus on the molecular enzymology of the catalytic subunit *per se* and on the common structural determinants that may be present in the receptors and in the coupler and effector molecules.

Receptor microaggregation, patching, ligand internalization and hormone action

As an outgrowth of the mobile receptor model and largely as a consequence of the availability both of specific anti-insulin receptor antibodies and of highly fluorescent hormone probes, there has been change in emphasis, in terms of hormone action, away from the ligands themselves to a focus on the receptors. Most striking have been the observations that insulin receptor antibodies can mimic most, if not all, of the biological actions of insulin *in vitro* that can be attributed to the occupation of the insulin receptor by insulin[6,7]. Importantly, the intact antibody or the bivalent (Fab)$_2$ species possess insulin-like activity, whereas the monovalent species, Fab, that behaves as a competitive inhibitor of insulin action in adipocytes, is inactive; the Fab molecule can be rendered active in the presence of anti-immunoglobulin antibody. Thus, as is the case with antibodies, a clustering of insulin receptor appears necessary for cell activation; a similar situation appears to hold for the epidermal growth factor-urogastrone (EGF-URO) receptor[8]. However, it is important to note that antibodies directed against the EGF-URO receptor do not mimic the action of EGF-URO[9]. The clear implication of the biological activity of the insulin antireceptor antibodies is that the information for the bioresponse resides primarily in the receptor itself and not in the active ligand. The function of the ligand *per se* appears to be that of a trigger molecule that initiates the series of reactions in which the receptor participates; once the process is activated by the ligand, its continued presence is not required by the receptor for subsequent events. This situation provides a new avenue for the design of novel drugs that could potentially activate receptor-mediated processes by combining with non-recognition portions of the receptor.

Direct biochemical methods, using both ^{125}I-labeled and highly fluorescently-labeled derivatives of insulin and EGF-URO have demonstrated that these hormones bind initially to highly mobile (diffusible) receptors, that are initially diffusely distributed, but that rapidly coalesce sequentially into patches and caps that become internalized. Autoradiographic studies indicate that the internalized labeled ligand is associated with lysosome-like structures. As discussed elsewhere[3], it appears that for insulin and EGF-URO, the receptor patching and internalization process is distinct from the immediate events that lead to cell activation, even in the case of a response (e.g. DNA synthesis) that occurs long after the initial ligand–receptor interaction. Thus, in terms of the action of many neurotransmitters and hormones, future work will undoubtedly concentrate on the initial rapid 'microaggregation' process, most likely involved in membrane activation. In this context, observations such as EGF-URO-modulated membrane phosphorylation (the receptor itself is possibly a kinase[10]), nicotinic cholinergic receptor phosphorylation, and the possible participation of the fatty acid cyclo-oxygenase system in the action of interferon[11] take on added significance.

It should also be pointed out, however, that for certain hormones, ligand internalization, subsequent to membrane binding, may play an important role. For instance, nerve growth factor (NGF) can be detected in the cell nucleus subsequent to binding at cell-surface receptor sites. Moreover, while controversial, data indicate that binding sites for insulin can be detected in isolated nuclei. Thus, although internalized hormone may not be required for cell activation (in the case of NGF, it has been demonstrated that 'non-leaky' sepharose-NGF derivatives lead to nerve cell differentiation), the internalized hormone fragments may play a unique role (e.g. control of receptor biosynthesis), separate from the cell activation process. Thus, future work might profitably examine the control, by internalized hormone, of processes other than cell stimulation.

Hormone-receptor mechanisms and the immune response

For some time, there has been a most fruitful interchange between those studying antibody-directed cell activation and those studying hormone-receptor mechanisms. In a sense, both the hormone receptors and antibody molecules are responsible both for a recognition function and a subsequent cell activation process. One attractive hypothesis[12] is that antibodies may have evolved from membrane-localized receptor molecules. Undoubtedly, the observed mobility of cell-associated antibodies and antigenic determinants had a large impact on the conceptualization of the mobile receptor model of hormone action. Recent direct observations of the lateral mobility of hormone receptors using fluorescent polypeptide derivatives, and of the apparent necessity of receptor clustering (insulin and EGF-URO) for cell activation strengthen the functional parallel that can be drawn between antibodies and receptors. Thus, it is very possible that the mechanisms responsible for the patching, capping, internalization and shedding of lymphocyte cell-surface antigen recognition molecules may be very similar to the analogous processes described[1] for hormone receptors. The implication would be that hormone receptors and cell-surface antibodies might have structural elements in common. In this regard, it is interesting that it has been previously suggested[13] that the C-regions of antibody molecules could serve as a 'handle', whereby molecules with differing specificities could be appropriately positioned in the membrane. As discussed above[1], there is a likelihood that receptors of a given class (e.g. those that modulate the adenylate cyclase system) may have molecular regions (? akin to the C-regions of antibodies) in common. It is striking in this regard that the recent structural data emerging for the insulin receptor[1] point to a four-chain oligomer of the type $(\alpha\beta)_2$, linked by disulphide bridges, very reminiscent of the immunoglobulin structure; very recent work with the receptor for basic-somatomedin suggests a structure closely related to the insulin receptor[14]. Possibly a similar kind of receptor 'family' relationship (isoreceptors) may be found between the structures of the various Fc receptors with different immunoglobulin specificities[15]. In future work, it will thus be of particular interest to look for structural elements in common both between receptors of a given class and between receptors and antibodies, for those regions of the molecules anchored in the cell membrane. In summary, it is quite likely that those mechanisms and structures involved in the activation of cells *via* the immune system may have common counterparts in the processes of hormone-directed cell activation. Given the remarkable advances in the molecular biology and methodology related to antibody synthesis and function, one can anticipate more exciting and fruitful interactions between the fields of immunology and receptor pharmacology.

Models for hormone-mediated cell activation

From the information presented above and in my companion article[1], it is possible to synthesize tentative models for four distinct reaction mechanisms that lead to receptor-modulated cell activation (Fig. 1). As outlined above, the receptors (R) for those hormones like glucagon (G) acting by adenylate cyclase activation, interact via a GTP-binding regulatory subunit (N-subunit) to modulate the activity of the catalytic (C) subunit. In Fig. 1A it is suggested that a receptor region (region 2), that may be similar in a variety of cyclase-related hormone receptors, interacts directly with the N-subunit. Further, the receptor is illustrated as having an internalization-related region (region 1) in common with a variety of receptors (Fig. 1B and D); interaction of region 1 with elements of the 'coated pit' area is presumed to be involved in the internalization process but not in the cell activation event. In Fig. 1A, the catalytic subunit of cyclase is shown to have a region (region 3) for interacting with a specific portion of the regulatory subunit; evidence suggests a conservation of this region between cell types and between species. In addition, a site on the catalytic subunit is shown (region 4) that might permit inhibitory regulation by a receptor like the one for insulin (Fig. 1B).

Very recent work suggests that insulin (I, Fig. 1) may act, in part, via the liberation of an intracellular peptide mediator generated by proteolysis of a membrane protein (MP)[16]. In the model for insulin action (Fig. 1B, essentially as proposed by Czech[16]), the disulphide-stabilized oligomeric insulin receptor ($\alpha_2\beta_2$, as reviewed previously[1,16]) is shown to be bivalent; a receptor area related to receptor internalization (region 1) and a region (region 4) for the interaction with a membrane glycoprotein receptor affinity regulator (GPR) are depicted. As suggested above, an area like region 4 might also play a role in the modulation of the catalytic subunit of adenylate cyclase. It is suggested (Fig. 1B) that receptor clustering (possibly involved in insulin-induced membrane potential changes) leads to the activation of a membrane protease that liberates a peptide mediator of insulin action (a phosphatase activator). The role of the peptide released from membranes by insulin stimulation is presently under intensive study.

In the case of the nicotinic receptor for acetylcholine (A, Fig. 1; reviewed briefly in my companion article[1]), cell stimulation is mediated by activation of an ion channel (Fig. 1C). Interestingly, this cholinergic receptor is thought to be bivalent, like the insulin receptor. It is believed that two receptor oligomers, linked in tandem by a disulphide bond, form a functional unit.

In contrast to the receptors for insulin and acetylcholine, the EGF-URO receptor appears to be a single-chain species. The receptor (Fig. 1D) is depicted to have the common internalization site (region 1) alluded to above. In addition, although very cautiously dealt with by Cohen and collaborators[10], it is suggested that the receptor possesses an intracellular catalytic site responsible for the phosphorylation of membrane protein tyrosine residues. It is quite possible that the phosphorylation reaction represents a first step in EGF-URO action. Although the phosphorylation reaction can proceed in detergent solution, it is uncertain whether or not receptor clustering is a prerequisite for the EGF-URO-stimulated enzymatic activity.

Thus, four distinct reaction pathways (cyclase activation and cAMP-modulated kinase activity; activation of membrane protease to liberate a peptide regulator; activation of ion transport; and intrinsic receptor kinase activity, leading to membrane constituent phosphorylation) appear to lead to cell activation. It is important to re-emphasize that, in keeping with the mobile receptor model[2,3], any particular

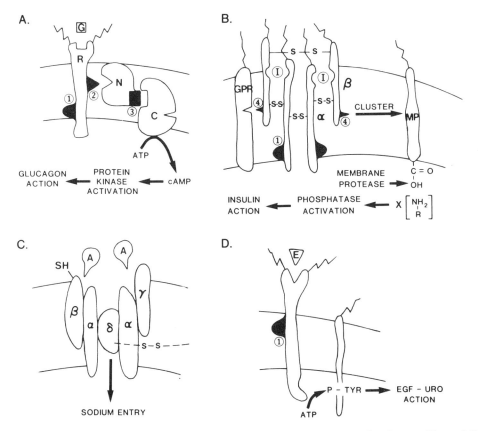

Fig. 1. Hypothetical models of hormone receptor-mediated cell activation. Receptors for glucagon (G, panel A), insulin (I, panel B), acetylcholine (A, panel C) and epidermal growth factor-urogastrone (E, panel D) are shown as integral membrane glycoproteins (oligosaccharide constituents:⋀⋀) that traverse the plasma membrane. Common receptor regions that relate to receptor function are depicted schematically: region 1 is involved in receptor internalization; regions 2 and 3 are related to the coupling of hormone receptor occupation to cyclase activation. Region 4 on the insulin receptor is shown to interact with a ligand affinity regulator glycoprotein (GPR); an analogous region may possibly interact with the catalytic subunit of cyclase. The four distinct activation mechanisms are discussed in the text. Panel A: G, glucagon; R, glucagon receptor; N, cyclase regulatory subunit; C, cyclase catalytic subunit; ATP, adenosine-5'-triphosphate; cAMP, cyclic adenosine 3'-5' monophosphate; Panel B: I, insulin; α, β, subunits of insulin receptor; GPR, glycoprotein regulator of insulin receptor affinity; MP, membrane protein substrate of insulin-mediated proteolytic activity; X, peptide mediator of insulin action; Panel C: A, acetylcholine; α, β, γ, δ, subunits of nicotinic acetylcholine receptor; Panel D: E, epidermal growth factor-urogastrone (EGF-URO); P-Tyr, phosphotyrosine. Disulphide bonds that link receptor oligomers are shown -S-S-, as is a free sulfhydryl (SH) on the acetylcholine receptor.

receptor oligomer could possibly modulate a number of such reaction pathways. Therefore, it may be inappropriate to attempt to identify a *single* reaction pathway as *the* primary event in the action of a particular hormone. Rather, the challenge in the future is to identify the matrix of concurrent receptor-modulated membrane-localized reactions that are involved in cell activation.

Receptors and disease

It is most rewarding that advances in receptor-related research have led to a better understanding of the pathophysiology of a variety of disease entities[16,17]. In a number of instances, the pathology appears to reside not in the receptor *per se*, but rather in the presence of autoantibodies that can interact with the receptor either as a competitive antagonist or as an agonist. Diseases in which antireceptor antibodies play a role are: Graves disease (receptor for thyroid stimulating hormone), myasthenia gravis (nicotinic receptor for acetylcholine), the syndrome of acanthosis nigricans Type B with insulin resistance (insulin receptor) and a population of patients exhibiting β-adrenergic hyporesponsiveness (β-receptor)[18]. It is of interest that this latter group of patients have been discovered as a result of a deliberate search for antibodies directed against the β-adrenergic receptor; evidence suggests that the circulating antibodies act as competitive inhibitors of isoproterenol action[18]. Thus, it would appear fruitful in any instance of a disease exhibiting either hormone resistance or the symptoms of hormone hyper-responsiveness to hunt for the presence of auto-antibodies directed against the receptor for the hormone of interest.

Aside from antireceptor antibodies, defects in the receptor system itself can lead to cellular malfunction. For instance, in type II hypercholesterolemia, there is a genetically determined defect in the acceptor* for low density lipoprotein (LDL) responsible for the cellular uptake of LDL-associated cholesterol[19]. At least two kinds of defects are known, one relating to an absolute deficiency of receptors and a second manifested by a defective internalization mechanism. In a variant of pseudohypoparathyroidism, it appears that the defect does not reside in the parathyroid hormone (PTH) receptor itself, but in another component of the receptor–effector system. The lack of cellular response has been attributed to a defect in the subunit (guanine nucleotide-binding or N-subunit) responsible for coupling receptor occupation to the activation of adenylate cyclase[20]. The essence of the above discussion is, that as more details become available concerning the multiple membrane-localized steps leading from receptor occupation to cell activation, the more likely it is that certain of the receptor system components will be found to play a role in the pathophysiology of certain diseases. It is thus pleasing to note that the in-depth study of receptor-related mechanisms is of particular interest and importance not only to the molecular biologist, but also to the entire biomedical community at large.

* The term acceptor, rather than receptor is used to denote the recognition–translocation function that is distinct from the recognition–stimulus function of 'traditional' receptors.

Reading list

1 Hollenberg, M. D. (1981) *Trends Pharmacol. Sci.* 2, 320–323
2 Cuatrecasas, P. and Hollenberg, M. D. (1976) *Adv. Protein Chem.* 30, 251–451
3 Hollenberg, M. D. (1979) *Pharmacol. Rev.* 30, 393–410
4 *Trends Pharmacol. Sci.* (1980) Vol. 9, pp. XI–XIV
5 Jakobs, K. H. and Schultz, G. (1980) *Trends Pharmacol. Sci.* 1, 331–333
6 Kahn, C. R., Baird, K. L., Flier, J. S., Grunfeld, C., Harmon, J. I., Harrison, L. C., Karlsson, F. A., Kasuga, M., King, G. L., Lang, U. C., Podskalny, J. M. and van Obberghen, E. (1981) *Recent Prog. Horm. Res.* 37, 477–538

7 Jacobs, S., Chang, K.-J. and Cuatrecasas, P. (1978) *Science* 200, 1283–1284
8 Schechter, Y., Hernaez, L., Schlessinger, J. and Cuatrecasas, P. (1979) *Nature (London)*, 278, 835–838
9 Haigler, H. and Carpenter, G. (1980) *Biochim. Biophys. Acta*, 598, 314–325
10 Cohen, S., Carpenter, G. and King, L., Jr. (1980) *J. Biol. Chem.* 255, 4834–4842
11 Pottathil, R., Chandrabose, K. A., Cuatrecasas, P. and Lang, D. J. (1980) *Proc. Natl Acad. Sci. U.S.A.* 77, 5437–5440
12 Dreyer, W. J., Gray, W. R., and Hood, L. (1967) *Cold Spring Harbor Symp. Quant. Biol.* 32, 353–367
13 Hood, L. and Prahl, J. (1971) *Adv. Immunol.* 14, 291–351
14 Hollenberg, M. D., Maturo, J. M. III and Bhaumick, B. in *Current Views on Insulin Receptors*, Proc. 1st Int. Symp. on Insulin Receptors, Rome, Sept. 1980 (Andreani, D. and DePirro, R., eds), Academic Press, New York (in press)
15 Mellman, I. S., Steinman, R. M., Unkeless, J. C. and Cohn, Z. A. (1980) *J. Cell Biol.* 86, 712–722
16 Czech, M. (1981) *Am. J. Med.* 70, 142–150
17 Jacobs, S. and Cuatrecasas, P. (1977) *N. Engl. J. Med.* 297, 1383–1386
18 Fraser, C. M., Harrison, L. C., Kaliner, M. C. and Venter, J. C. (1980) *Clin. Res.* 28, 236A
19 Anderson, R. G. W., Goldstein, J. L. and Brown, M. S. (1977) *Nature (London)*, 270, 695–699
20 Farfel, Z., Buckman, A. S., Kaslow, H. R., Brothers, V. M. and Bourne, H. R. (1980) *N. Engl. J. Med.* 303, 237–242

Activation and inhibition of adenylate cyclase by hormones: mechanistic aspects

Alexander Levitzki

Department of Biological Chemistry, The Hebrew University of Jerusalem, 91904 Jerusalem, Israel.

Eucaryotic adenylate cyclases are coupled to hormone and neurotransmitter receptors in two modes: stimulatory and inhibitory. Stimulation of cyclase by agonist requires the presence of GTP at a concentration range of 0.01–0.10 μM. Hormone-induced inhibition of adenylate cyclase requires GTP at a concentration range of 0.2–6.0 μM. The possible modes of coupling between the stimulatory receptor, the GTP regulatory protein and the catalytic unit have been examined in the light of accumulating experimental data. It is concluded that the main event in the activation of the enzyme is the bimolecular encounter between the agonist-receptor complex and the complex between the GTP regulatory site and the catalytic moiety. An analysis of existing knowledge about the mode of inhibition of adenylate cyclase by hormones suggests that the inhibitory hormone functions through a separate GTP binding site which either interacts directly with the catalytic unit or uncouples the stimulatory GTP site from the catalytic site.

Introduction

Hormone-dependent adenylate cyclases are composed of three functional units: the receptor which binds the hormone or neurotransmitter, R, the GTP regulatory protein, N (or G/F), and the catalytic moiety, C. Upon agonist binding to R and of GTP to N, C is activated and is converted from its inactive form to an active one, catalysing the conversion of ATP to cAMP and pyrophosphate. A large variety of agonists were found to activate adenylate cyclase. These include small molecules such as l-epinephrine, histamine and serotonin, small peptides such as vaso-intestinal peptide (VIP), and large polypeptide hormones such as glucagon, ACTH and TSH. The different receptors differ in their binding specificity, as can easily be concluded from these abbreviated lists, but seem to activate the adenylate cyclase moiety by a similar or even identical mechanism. Indeed, it has been shown that different receptors from different cells can hybridize with the same adenylate cyclase system that possesses intact N and C. For example, β-adrenergic receptors can be transferred from the turkey erythrocyte into Friend erythroleukemia cells and activate the adenylate cyclase of the latter[1]. Similarly, the glucagon receptor from rat liver membranes can also be implanted into Friend erythroleukemia cells and activate its adenylate cyclase[2].

Kinetic evidence supports the view that different receptors in the *same cell* couple to a single pool of adenylate cyclase. For example, adenosine receptors of the type

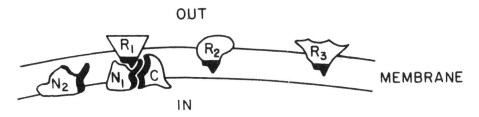

Fig. 1. The interaction between R, N and C. Receptors for different hormones (R_1 and R_2) probably possess identical interaction domains with different N units. Similarly, different N units from different sources most probably possess similar protein domains for interaction with different C units. Therefore, it follows that different cyclases possess common structural features for interaction with different N-units.

A2 and β-adrenergic receptors in turkey erythrocytes are coupled to the same pool of adenylate cyclase[3].

Similarly, the N unit also seems to be universal, namely, it can couple to a variety of C units from different sources. For example, AC⁻ S49 lymphoma cells possess β-adrenergic receptors and an intact C unit, but lack a functional N unit. Restoration of a functional β-receptor-dependent adenylate cyclase can be achieved by an N unit supplied by a large variety of cells such as wild type S49 lymphoma cells[4], rabbit livers[5] and turkey erythrocytes[6].

These findings indicate that different receptors must possess similar or identical protein domains which interact with the N unit, and that different N units possess similar or identical domains which interact with the same domain on the C unit (Fig. 1).

Direct structural information

(i) *The receptor.* Direct structural information on the receptor-dependent adenylate cyclase system is still scarce. Among the receptors linked to adenylate cyclase, the β-adrenergic receptor system provides most of the currently-known information. The β-receptor from frog erythrocytes has been purified and its subunit mol. wt was found to be 58,000[7]. The β-receptor subunit of the turkey erythrocyte has been shown to possess a mol. wt of 37-41,000[8]. The lubrol-PX solubilized β-receptor from S49 cells possesses a mol. wt of 74,000[9], where the subunit mol. wt of this receptor is not known. Most probably the receptor in lubrol is in its oligomeric state. The mol. wt of gonadotropin receptor is 160,000, which strongly indicates that it is composed of subunits[10,11]. Clearly, much more work is needed to establish the structure of these receptors. So far, even less is known about the structure of other receptors linked to adenylate cyclase.

(ii) *The N unit.* The N binding protein in its native state is oligomeric with a mol. wt of 90–130,000[4]. Aside from the 42,000 mol. wt subunit, a subunit of about 55,000 mol. wt has been identified and was found to be a substrate for ADP-ribosylation.

The N unit is composed of two to three types of subunits. One of these subunits possesses a mol. wt of 42,000[12] and is the substrate of the cholera toxin catalysed ADP-ribosylation[13,14]. It is also believed that this subunit possesses the hormone-dependent GTPase activity linked to the adenylate cyclase system (see below). It has recently been suggested that the state of aggregation of the N unit depends on the presence of guanyl nucleotides. Thus, binding of the GTP analog GTPγS induces a reduction in the molecular weight of the N binding protein, most probably down to the activated 42K unit[15].

(iii) *The C unit.* The catalytic unit which is associated with hormone-dependent cyclase has not yet been purified. The high molecular weights reported for detergent solubilized adenylate cyclases, however, may be taken as an indication of their oligomeric nature (Ref. 16 and citations therein).

In summary, the available structural information is still limited, and much more work is needed in order to achieve a more complete structural description of the system.

Mechanistic aspects

The current views on the mode of action of hormone-dependent adenylate cyclase are summarized in Fig. 2. Both hormone binding to R and GTP binding to N are required to induce activation of C to the cAMP producing state. The active state of the system decays concomitantly with the hydrolysis of GTP to GDP and Pi at the N regulatory site. Replenishment of N with GTP and the continued presence of hormone at the receptor assures the ability of the system to re-acquire its active cAMP producing state. This 'on–off' cycle with its GTPase element (Fig. 2) is the accepted dogma that accounts well for most of the properties of hormone-dependent adenylate cyclase. We shall list a few:

(i) Hormone dependent adenylate cyclases also possess hormone dependent GTPase activity. Indeed, this activity, first shown in β-receptor dependent turkey ery-

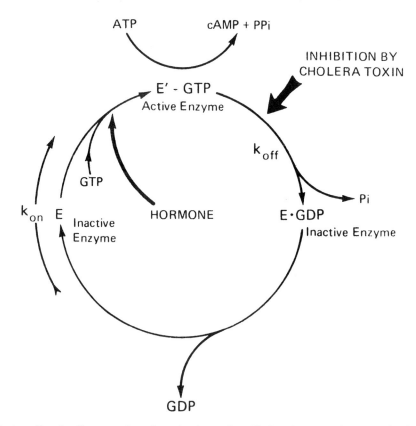

Fig. 2. The 'on-off' cycle of hormone dependent adenylate cyclase. The inactive enzyme is converted to its active form upon the synergistic action of the stimulatory hormone and the replacement of GDP with GTP. The process of this conversion is first order and is characterized by the first order rate constant k_{on}. The cAMP producing state $E'\cdot GTP$ decays to the inactive state concomitantly with the hydrolysis of GTP at the N-regulatory unit. The GTPase turn-off reaction is again a first order decay process, characterized by the constant k_{off}. This GTPase step is blocked by the cholera toxin catalysed ADP-ribosylation of the 42,000 mol. wt subunit within the N-unit. The function of the hormone is most probably limited to catalyse the conformational transition of the inactive enzyme to its active form, and is not involved in catalysing the release of GDP or the insertion of GTP (see text).

throcyte adenylate cyclase[17], has since been demonstrated in a glucagon-dependent cyclase[18], a pancreozymin-dependent cyclase[19], and a prostaglandin E_1-dependent cyclase[20].

(ii) The use of non-hydrolysable GTP analogs should increase adenylate cyclase activity. Indeed, in the presence of GppNHp, GppCH$_2$p, or GTPγS, a high activity form of cyclase is obtained in many systems[16,21-23,36]. In the presence of these analogs, the enzyme is 'trapped' in a persistently active form due to the complete blockade of the 'turn-off' reaction.

(iii) Direct inhibition of the GTPase reaction by 'ADP-ribosylation' catalysed by cholera toxin induces activation of the cyclase[20,24-27]. Indeed, this is expected according to the 'on-off' model (Fig. 2). The slow-down in the 'off' GTPase reaction should elevate the steady state concentration of active cyclase in the presence of GTP. This covalent interconversion occurs at the N unit, specifically at the 42,000 mol. wt subunit, which may indeed be the site for the GTPase activity. So far, attempts to demonstrate GTPase activity of the isolated and purified N unit have not been successful. It is, however, feasible that N has *no* GTPase activity in the *absence of an agonist–receptor complex*.

(iv) From the quantitative measurements of the rate of enzyme activation by hormone and guanyl nucleotide (the 'on' reaction) and the decay of the cAMP producing state to the basal state (the 'off' reaction), one should be able to compute the *fraction* of the total pool of cyclase which is in the active state in the presence of GTP. Such measurements have been conducted[23-25,28-29] and, in fact, demonstrated that the two-state model presented in Fig. 2 is sufficient to account for the 'on-off' cycle.

Measuring the 'on' reaction

The process of cyclase activation can be monitored with relative ease[28,29] because non-hydrolysable GTP analogs such as GppNHp or GTPγS can be used. Under these conditions, the 'off' reaction does not take place and, therefore, does not 'mess up' the kinetics. In the presence of such an analog every adenylate cyclase molecule that is converted to its active form is 'stuck' in this state, since the hydrolysis step cannot take place. Thus, the *entire population* of enzyme molecules is converted to the active form which is now 'permanent' or 'persistent'. The kinetics of this process is first order and has been analysed in great detail in the turkey erythrocyte system[28-32].

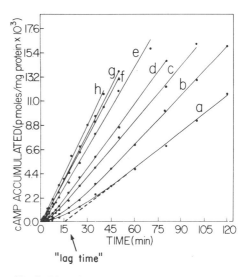

Fig. 3. The calculation of k_{on}. The accumulation of cAMP is given by equation 2, as shown in the text. At long time intervals ($t \to \infty$), the exponential term $e^{-k_{on}t}$ approaches zero and the straight line which now describes the production of cAMP will be given by the equation: $cAMP_t = V_{max}t - \frac{V_{max}}{k_{on}}$. Clearly, the intercept of the straight line at the time axis ($cAMP_t = 0$) occurs when $t = \frac{1}{k_{on}}$. Thus, the value of k_{on} can be obtained graphically or by a best fit to equation 2. Indeed, the two procedures have been used by us to obtain a substantial number of k_{on} values[28-32]. The data in this figure are taken from Ref. 30; the time course of cAMP production by l-epinephrine dependent cyclase has been measured in turkey erythrocytes treated with cis-vaccenic acid at 25°C. Increasing the amount of cis-vaccenic acid incorporated into the membrane (from a to h, a = control, with no cis-vaccenic acid), was found to increase the rate of enzyme activation (k_{on}), namely, to shorten the lag time, as is seen in the figure[30].

It was found that the process can be described by the equation:

$$\frac{V_{max}}{V_{max} - V_t} = k_{on} \times t, \quad (1)$$

a typical expression for a first order process. V_t is the specific activity at any given time, t, and V_{max} is the maximal specific activity attainable with the non-hydrolysable GTP analog. The integrated form of the equation is[29]:

$$cAMP_t = V_{max} t + \frac{V_{max}}{k_{on}} (e^{-k_{on}t} - 1). \quad (2)$$

Hence, following the production of cAMP as a function of time, yields a curve with a 'lag time', the length of which depends on k_{on}, namely, on the rate of conversion of the inactive enzyme to the active enzyme. Obviously, after 'enough' time, the value $k_{on}t$ becomes large, the exponential term 'disappears', and a straight line is obtained (Fig. 3). This occurs when all the cyclase molecules have been converted to their activated state. Extrapolation of the straight line back to the time ordinate yields the characteristic 'lag time' which is related to k_{on} simply by a reciprocal, namely,

$$k_{on} = \frac{1}{t_{lag}} \text{(see Fig. 3).} \quad (3)$$

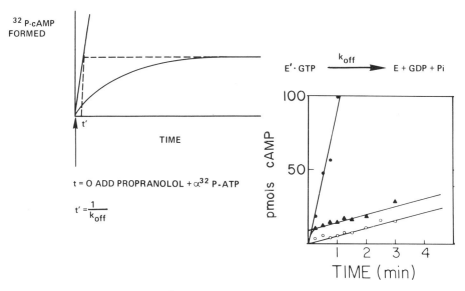

Fig. 4. The measurement of k_{off}. Two identical adenylate cyclase systems are allowed to produce non-radioactive cAMP in the presence of agonist, GTP and non-radioactive substrate ATP. At time zero, one system receives an antagonist or GDPβS with [α-^{32}P]ATP and the control system only [α-^{32}P]ATP. From that time on the production of ^{32}P-cAMP of the experimental system will follow a first order decay process and will level off at a plateau typical to the basal activity of the system. The control system produces a linear time course of ^{32}P-cAMP production. The extrapolation of the plateau back to the control line yields k_{off}. The equation characterizing the production of ^{32}P-cAMP is $cAMP_t = \frac{V_{max}}{k_{off}} (1 - exp(-k_{off}t))$, where at $t \to \infty$, $[cAMP]_{TOTAL} = \frac{V_{max}}{k_{off}}$. The control system produces ^{32}P-cAMP according to $cAMP_t = V_{max}t$. At time t', the control system produces the maximal amount of ^{32}P-cAMP yielded by the decaying system, namely, $V_{max}t' = \frac{V_{max}}{k_{off}}$. Thus, k_{off} is read directly from the graph. Again, the more accurate determination is by a computer fit to the full equation, as previously described[29,31].

Inset (right): Turkey erythrocyte membranes (6.25 mg ml^{-1}) were incubated at 37°C with 0.3 mM ATP, 4 mM MgCl$_2$, 50 mM Tris-HCl, pH 7.4, 20 μM l-isoproterenol, 1.0 μM GTP, 0.4 mg theophylline, 1.0 mM creatine phosphate, and 7.5 units/assay of creatine kinase. At time zero, ethanol-free [α-^{32}P]ATP (200 cpm pmol^{-1}) were added with (▲) or without (●) dl-propranolol (0.5 mM final concentration). A control experiment with no agonist was run in parallel (○). At different times, 100 μl samples were removed to a stopping solution containing 2% sodium dodecyl sulfate and then analysed for ^{32}P-cAMP.

Thus, the experimental measurement of k_{on} is an easy task. A more accurate way to obtain k_{on} is, of course, by the computer fit of the data to equation 2.

Measuring the 'off' reaction

The measurement of the 'off' reaction proved to be more tricky as k_{off} proved to be much faster than k_{on}. Two methods, which are essentially one, are in use. The cyclase is allowed to operate with agonist, GTP and non-radioactive substrate (ATP); at time zero, an antagonist is added in excess amounts. Thus, all receptors become occupied with an antagonist in a diffusion-controlled time scale (microseconds) and the cyclase cannot be reactivated. Simultaneously with the antagonist, $[\alpha\text{-}^{32}P]ATP$ is added. Thus, at zero time, the fraction of cyclase molecules that are in the active state decays to zero in a first order process, where the characteristic rate constant is k_{off}. Following the time course of ^{32}P-cAMP production from the time the antagonist and $[\alpha\text{-}^{32}P]ATP$ are added, yields the value of k_{off}[24-25,29,31]. A simpler graphical method can also be used (see Fig. 4). When a hormone antagonist is not available, GDPβS, a GTP antagonist[33,34], can be used with the achievement of the same phenomenology.

Is the 'on–off' description sufficient?

In one system, the β-adrenergic receptor dependent adenylate cyclase of turkey erythrocytes, the full analysis of k_{on}, k_{off}, and their relationship has been performed[17,23-25,28-34]. The 'on–off' cycle predicts that the fraction of active cyclase at any given time will be:

$$\frac{[E']}{[E_0]} = \frac{k_{on}}{k_{on} + k_{off}}. \quad (4)$$

As $\frac{[E']}{[E_0]}$ equals $\frac{V_{max}^{GTP}}{V_{max}^{GppNHp}}$, where V_{max}^{GTP} is the maximal hormone dependent cyclase activity in the presence of GTP, and V_{max}^{GppNHp} is the maximal specific activity in the presence of GppNHp, equation 4 can be rewritten as follows:

$$\frac{V_{max}^{GTP}}{V_{max}^{GppNHp}} = \frac{k_{on}}{k_{on} + k_{off}}. \quad (5)$$

These four parameters can be and have been measured *independently* for a number of β-agonists. The quantitative fit was found to be excellent[29,31]. Furthermore, the inhibition of the hormone dependent GTPase activity by cholera toxin catalysed ADP-ribosylation is reflected in both a slower k_{off} and an increased value of V_{max}^{GTP}[24,25]. Indeed, when the cholera toxin-induced changes in V_{max}^{GTP} and in k_{off} are inserted into equation 5, the relationship (equation 5) is found to hold perfectly. It seems, therefore, that for the turkey erythrocyte system, the 'on–off' cycle, using a two-state model for the cyclase (Fig. 2), is sufficient for a full description of the system.

Apparent discrepancies

The 'on–off' cycle, as formulated (Fig. 2, equation 5), predicts that the GTP dependence of the hormone-dependent adenylate cyclase and of the coupled GTPase activity should be *identical*. However, in two systems, i.e. the β-receptor-dependent adenylate cyclase[35] and the PGE$_1$-dependent cyclase of human platelets[20], a large discrepancy between the GTP dependence of cyclase and that of its coupled GTPase could be identified (Table I).

TABLE I. The GTP dependence of hormone-dependent cyclase and hormone-dependent GTPase

System	Km for GTP (μM)		Refs.
	Cyclase	GTPase	
Turkey erythrocyte	0.014	0.2	35,17
Human platelet	0.04	0.6	20

A small modification of the classical model described in Fig. 2 can, however, take care of this discrepancy. For example, if one assumes that the enzyme

$$E + GTP \underset{k_2}{\overset{k_1}{\rightleftharpoons}} \underset{\text{Cyclase active}}{E' \cdot GTP} \underset{k_4}{\overset{k_3}{\rightleftharpoons}} \underset{\text{GTPase active}}{E'' \cdot GTP} \qquad (6)$$
$$\overset{k_5}{\rightarrow} E + GDP + Pi$$

exists in a cyclase-active state $E' \cdot GTP$ and a GTPase active state $E'' \cdot GTP$, one obtains that $K_m^{\text{cyclase}} < K_m^{\text{GTPase}}$, if $k_3 > k_4 + k_5$. Clearly, refinements of the 'classical' 'on–off' model require a more thorough investigation in order to clearly define the correct modification needed.

GDP-release

It has often been suggested that the rate-limiting step to adenylate cyclase activation may be the removal of GDP from the N regulatory site, since the latter must be removed before activation can take place[28,36–38]. Experimental attempts to demonstrate that GDP release is indeed rate limiting[39], were shown to be inadequate[40]. The total removal of bound GDP from turkey erythrocyte adenylate cyclase, however[32], was found not to alter the kinetics of hormone plus GppNHp activation. Therefore, it seems that the release of GDP from its binding site is not the rate-limiting step. Nevertheless, the release of GDP from the site may occur *as soon as* the rate-limiting step takes place. This is a realistic possibility, since hormone-dependent GDP release has been demonstrated[41,42].

The catalytic role of the receptor and 'collision coupling'

In the attempt to explore in some detail the nature of the rate-limiting step in the overall process of turkey erythrocyte adenylate cyclase activation by hormone, an effort to dissect k_{on} was performed in the turkey erythrocyte β-receptor system[29,32]. It was found that k_{on} is a saturating function of hormone at all concentrations of guanyl nucleotide (GppNHp). The value of k_{on} was found not to be dependent on GppNHp concentration at any nucleotide concentration[32]. These findings indicate that the hormone–receptor complex participates in the process of activation, where the apparent hormone–receptor dissociation constant elucidated from these measurements is identical to that obtained from direct binding measurements[29,32]. The absence of an effect of GppNHp concentration strongly indicates that the *binding of the nucleotide is not rate limiting* and, most probably, not a result of the interaction between the H·R complex with the N unit. Carrying this conclusion a step further, it could be stated that the binding of the regulatory ligands, hormone, and guanyl nucleotide (GTP or an analog) is random and independent[32].

Another set of experiments revealed that the role of the receptor is catalytic[29]. The progressive decrease in the number of β-adrenergic receptors on the turkey erythrocyte membranes, using a specific β-receptor-directed affinity label, reduced the *rate* of cyclase activation but not the maximal specific activity attainable with hormone and GppNHp. Thus, k_{on} was found to be *linearly dependent* on receptor concentration:

$$k_{on} = k_{on(\text{intrinsic})}[R_T]. \qquad (7)$$

This surprising result led to the formulation of the 'collision coupling' model[29,43] in which it is assumed that the hormone–receptor complex makes a transient encounter with the adenylate cyclase complex:

$$H \cdot R + N_{GTP} \cdot C \quad \{H \cdot R \cdot N_{GTP} \cdot C$$
$$H \cdot R \cdot N'_{GTP} \cdot C'\} \rightarrow HR + N'_{GTP} \cdot C'$$
$$N'_{GTP} \cdot C' \rightarrow N \cdot C + GDP + Pi. \qquad (8)$$

The intermediate (in brackets), according to this model, does not accumulate.

This formulation accounts well for the data, since it predicts: (i) strict first order kinetics of cyclase activation by hormone and GppNHp; (ii) a linear dependence of the rate constant of activation, k_{on}, on receptor concentration; and (iii) a Michaelian (non-cooperative) dependence of k_{on} on the hormone concentration, yielding the same hormone-receptor dissociation constant as binding experiments. Similar results were obtained for the activation of adenylate cyclase by glucagon and GppNHp in the rat liver system[44]. In that system it was found that the reduction in the concentration of glucagon receptor also reduced the rate of enzyme activation but not the maximal specific activity attainable with glucagon and GppNHp.

Criticism of the 'collision coupling' model

Some workers have raised certain objections concerning the 'collision coupling' mechanism. For example, it was argued that since GTP induces a decrease in β-receptor affinity towards β-agonists, it must mean that any mechanism has to incorporate within it a long-lived complex between the receptor and the guanyl nucleotide binding protein[45,46]. Unfortunately, in the frog system[46] where such GTP effects were found on the β-receptor, detailed kinetic experiments have not been performed. In the turkey erythrocyte system we have recently performed very detailed experiments on the effect of

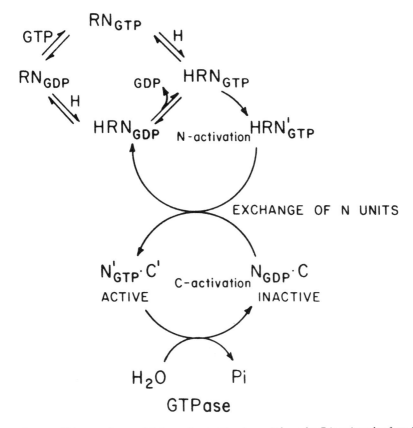

Fig. 5. The exchange collision coupling model. According to this scheme, N bound to R is activated to form N'_{GTP}, once hormone binds to R and GTP becomes accessible. The R bound N'_{GTP} unit now exchanges with the N_{GDP} or empty N which is bound to the catalytic unit C. C becomes activated and the cycle repeats itself. The essential element of the collision coupling, namely, the catalytic action of the receptor, is retained. This type of mechanism also allows for nucleotide effects on the receptor, as observed in numerous systems.

guanyl nucleotides on the affinity of β-agonists toward the receptor, using the new β-ligand [^{125}I]cyanopindolol (^{125}I-CYP). We have found[35] evidence for the nucleotide-induced shift. Still, it is feasible to reconcile the GTP-induced 'shift', which indicates that R and N can form a long-lived complex, with a 'collision coupling' type model (Fig. 5). In that modification of the 'collision coupling' model, one assumed that *both* the R unit and the C unit possess an N unit which are *exchanged* during the process of activation. So far this is the only model, among all N shuttle models (Fig. 6), which can account for all the experimental observations: (i) first order kinetics of activation; (ii) independence of the *rate* of cyclase activation (k_{on}) on the concentration of N units or on GppNHp; and (iii) a strictly linear dependence of the rate of activation (k_{on}) on receptor concentration.

Other 'N-shuttle' models

The ability of the hormone–receptor complex to activate N in the absence of an active C unit, where later the activated N'_{GppNHp} unit can confer activity to the cyclase of AC$^-$ S49 cells[45], the GTP-induced decrease in agonist affinity[46,47] brings about the suggestion that N 'shuttles' between R and C (model 4, Fig. 6). This model and similar models *cannot* account for the full kinetic picture of the native turkey erythrocyte β-receptor-dependent adenylate cyclase.

In a detailed analysis[32,48] it can be shown that an 'N-shuttle' model of this type leads to complex kinetic patterns of enzyme activation, which are not experimentally

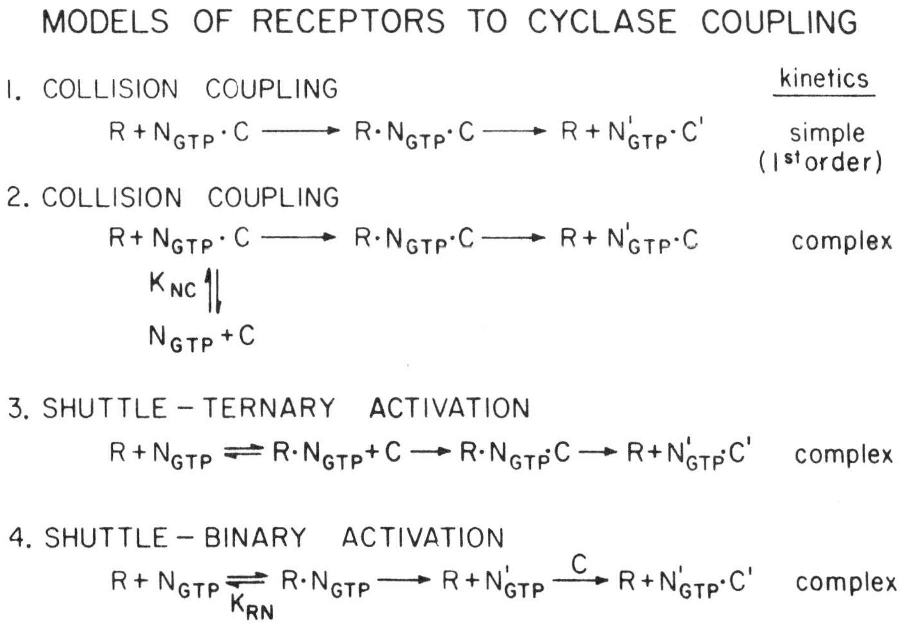

MODELS OF RECEPTORS TO CYCLASE COUPLING

                                                                                              kinetics

1. COLLISION COUPLING

   $R + N_{GTP} \cdot C \longrightarrow R \cdot N_{GTP} \cdot C \longrightarrow R + N'_{GTP} \cdot C'$ simple (1st order)

2. COLLISION COUPLING

   $R + N_{GTP} \cdot C \longrightarrow R \cdot N_{GTP} \cdot C \longrightarrow R + N'_{GTP} \cdot C$ complex

   $K_{NC} \updownarrow$

   $N_{GTP} + C$

3. SHUTTLE – TERNARY ACTIVATION

   $R + N_{GTP} \rightleftharpoons R \cdot N_{GTP} + C \longrightarrow R \cdot N_{GTP} \cdot C \longrightarrow R + N'_{GTP} \cdot C'$ complex

4. SHUTTLE – BINARY ACTIVATION

   $R + N_{GTP} \underset{K_{RN}}{\rightleftharpoons} R \cdot N_{GTP} \longrightarrow R + N'_{GTP} \xrightarrow{C} R + N'_{GTP} \cdot C'$ complex

Fig. 6. N-shuttle models. The original 'collision coupling' model and N-shuttle models are depicted in the figure. The collision coupling model predicts simple first order kinetics of cyclase activation by hormone and GppNHp. All other models which allow N to be activated first by R and then migrate to C, activating the latter, predict complex kinetic patterns (models 3 and 4). Even when one allows N to dissociate from C in an essentially 'collision coupling' type mechanism, a complex kinetic pattern is observed. A very detailed analysis of these and other derived models[32,48] reveals that in order to account for the experimental observations in the turkey erythrocyte systems, one must reject N-shuttle models altogether, except for the model described in Fig. 5.

observed in the native turkey erythrocyte system. The 'collision coupling' model in which N units can be exchanged between the R unit and the C unit (Fig. 5), is the only shuttle type model that is compatible with the experimental results. Clearly, the last word on this issue has not yet been said, and more experimental work is needed to clarify these details.

An appealing aspect of the model described in Fig. 5 is that it allows for effects of guanyl nucleotides on the receptor, which are separate from the effects on cyclase. For example, at high concentrations of GTP, far above those which saturate the activation cycles in Fig. 1 or 5, all of the GDP in the system may be replaced by GTP. Under such conditions, the receptor interacts with a nucleotide binding protein to which only GTP is bound at all times. This receptor may therefore exhibit a low affinity towards the agonist as compared to receptor which interacts with N_{GDP} or N_{empty}. This may occur either because N_{GTP} tends to dissociate from R altogether, or because it induces a conformational change at the R unit, although remaining bound to the latter.

Inhibition of adenylate cyclase by inhibitory hormones

In recent years it has been shown that certain hormones induce the inhibition of adenylate cyclase[49-57]. In all of these cases it is established that the inhibition requires GTP at concentrations from 5 to 20-fold higher than those needed to induce cyclase activation. This finding by itself already indicates that the GTP site which mediates the effect of the inhibitory hormone may be *distinct* from the GTP site which mediates the activation of hormone (the GTPase site). Recently Koski and Klee[58] have shown that Na^+ inhibits a low K_m GTPase of neuroblastoma × glyoma NG-108-15 cells and that morphine and enkephalin, which inhibit cyclase in that system, reverse this Na^+-dependent GTPase inhibition. These data were taken to mean that the stimulation of the GTPase (increase in k_{off}) by the inhibitory hormone is the mechanism through which morphine and enkephalin inhibit the NG-108-15 adenylate cyclase, via the enkephalin receptor. Indeed, according to equation 5 and the scheme in Fig. 2, an increase of k_{off} should induce cyclase inhibition, if its numerical value is close to that of k_{on}.

In another system, however, the purified human platelet membranes system, we found[59] that the inhibitory hormone l-epinephrine operating through the α_2-adrenergic receptor *does not* affect either k_{off}, GTPase activity or k_{on}. Thus, we prefer the mechanism by which an inhibitory hormone inhibits cyclase, namely, through a *separate* GTP regulatory site, as suggested by Rodbell[22]. This inhibitory site may interact either *directly* with the catalytic unit or interfere in the interaction between the stimulatory N unit with C. In both cases the intrinsic properties of the stimulatory unit such as its hormone-dependent GTPase activity, remain unaffected. Indeed, α_2-adrenergic agonists fail to inhibit the PGE_1-dependent GTPase activity in purified human platelet membranes, whereas they inhibit effectively the PGE_1-dependent cyclase under the same conditions[20,59]. The seemingly contradictory observations in the NG-108-15 cells and in purified human platelet membranes only demonstrate the need for much more work in this field.

Acknowledgements

The experimental data from our laboratory were obtained from studies supported by NIH grants GM 26604 and GM 27087, as well as a grant from the Deutsche Forschungsgemeinschaft, and the U.S.–Israel Binational Research Foundation (BRF) Jerusalem, Israel.

Reading list

1 Schramm, M., Orly, J., Eimerl, S. and Korner, M. (1977) *Nature (London)* 268, 310–313
2 Schramm, M. (1979) *Proc. Natl Acad. Sci. U.S.A.* 76, 1174–1178

3. Tolkovsky, A. M. and Levitzki, A. (1978) *Biochemistry*, 17, 3811–3817
4. Ross, E. M. and Gilman, A. G. (1977) *Proc. Natl Acad. Sci. U.S.A.* 74, 3715–3719
5. Northup, J. K., Sternweis, P. C., Ross, E. M. and Gilman, A. G. (1980) *Proc. Natl Acad. Sci. U.S.A.* 77, 6516–6520
6. Hanski, E., Sternweis, P. C., Northup, J. K., Dromerick, A. W. and Gilman A. G. (1981) *J. Biol. Chem.*
7. Shorr, R. G., Lefkowitz, R. J. and Caron, M. G. (1981) *J. Biol. Chem.* 254, 5820–5826
8. Atlas, D. and Levitzki, A. (1978) *Nature (London)* 272, 370–371
9. Haga, T., Haga, K. and Gilman, A. G. (1977) *J. Biol. Chem.* 252, 5776–5782
10. Dufau, M. L., Chareau, E. H. and Catt, K. J. (1973) *J. Biol. Chem.* 248, 6973–6982
11. Dufau, M. L., Chareau, E. H., Ryan, D. and Catt, K. (1974) *FEBS Lett.* 39, 149–153
12. Pfeuffer, T. (1977) *J. Biol. Chem.* 252, 7224–7234
13. Gill, D. M. and Meren, R. (1978) *Proc. Natl Acad. Sci. U.S.A.* 75, 3050–3054
14. Cassel, D. and Pfeuffer, T. (1978) *Proc. Natl Acad. Sci. U.S.A.* 75, 2669–2773
15. Gilman, A. G., Stornweis, P. C., Northup, J. K., Hunski, E., Smigel, M. D. and Kohn, R. A. (1981) *J. Cyclic Nucl, Res,* (in press)
16. Ross, E. M. and Gilman, A. G. (1980) *Annu. Rev. Biochem.* 49, 533–563
17. Cassel, D. and Selinger, Z. (1976) *Biochim. Biophys. Acta* 452, 3829–3835
18. Kimura, N. and Shimada, N. (1980) *FEBS Lett.* 117, 172–174
19. Lambert, M., Svoboda, M. and Christophe, J. (1979) *FEBS Lett.* 99, 303–307
20. Lester, H., Steer, M. L. and Levitzki, A. (1982) *Proc. Natl Acad. Sci. U.S.A.* 79
21. Levitzki, A. and Helmreich, E. J. M. (1979) *FEBS Lett.* 10, 213–219
22. Rodbell, M. (1980) *Nature (London)* 284, 17–21
23. Levitzki, A. (1977) *Biochem. Biophys. Res. Commun.* 74, 1154–1159
24. Cassel, D. and Selinger, Z. (1977) *Proc. Natl Acad. Sci. U.S.A.* 74, 3307–3311
25. Cassel, D., Levkovitz, H. and Selinger Z. (1977) *J. Cyclic. Nucleotide. Res.* 3, 393–406
26. Ross, E. M., Maguire, M. E., Sturgill, T. W., Biltonen, T. W. and Gilman, A. G. (1977) *J. Biol. Chem.* 252, 5761–5775
27. Levinson, S. L. and Blume, A. J. (1977) *J. Biol. Chem.* 252, 3766–3774
28. Sevilla, N., Steer, M. L. and Levitzki, A. (1976) *Biochemistry*, 15, 3494–3499
29. Tolkovsky, A. M. and Levitzki, A. (1978) *Biochemistry*, 17, 3795–3810
30. Hanski, E., Rimon, G. and Levitzki, A. (1979) *Biochemistry*, 18, 846–853
31. Arad, H. and Levitzki, A. (1979) *Mol. Pharmacol.* 16, 748–756
32. Tolkovsky, A. M., Braun, S. and Levitzki, A. (1981) *Proc. Natl Acad. Sci. U.S.A.* (in press)
33. Eckstein, F., Cassel, D., Levkovitz, H., Lowe, M. and Selinger, Z. (1979) *J. Biol. Chem.* 254, 9829–9834
34. Cassel, D., Eckstein, F., Lowe, M. and Selinger, Z. (1979) *J. Biol. Chem.* 254, 9835–9838
35. Braun, S., Tolkovsky, A. M. and Levitzki, A. *EMBO J.* (in press)
36. Pfeuffer, T. and Helmreich, E. J. M. (1975) *J. Biol. Chem.* 250, 867–876
37. Blume, A. J. and Foster, C. J. (1976) *J. Biol. Chem.* 251, 3399–3404
38. Sevilla, N. and Levitzki, A. (1977) *FEBS Lett.* 78, 129–134
39. Swillens, S., Juvent, M. and Dumont, J. E. (1979) *FEBS Lett.* 108, 365–368
40. Levitzki, A. (1980) *FEBS Lett.* 115, 9–10
41. Cassel, D. and Selinger, Z. (1978) *Proc. Natl. Acad. Sci. U.S.A.* 75, 4155–4159
42. Pike, L. J. and Lefkowitz, R. J. (1981) *J. Biol. Chem.* 256, 2207–2212
43. Arad, H., Rimon, G. and Levitzki, A. (1981) *J. Biol. Chem.* 256, 1593–1597
44. Houslay, M. D., Dipple, I. and Elliott, K. R. F. (1980) *Biochem. J.* 186, 649–658
45. Citri, Y. and Schramm, M. (1980) *Nature (London)* 287, 297–300
46. DeLean, A., Stadel, J. M. and Lefkowitz, R. J. (1980) *J. Biol. Chem.* 255, 7108–7118
47. Maguire, M. E., Van Arsdale, P. M. and Gilman, A. G. (1976) *Mol. Pharmacol.* 12, 335–339
48. Tolkovsky, A. M. and Levitzki, A. (1981) *J. Cyclic Nucleotides.* 7(3), 139–150
49. Jakobs, K. H., Saur, W. and Schultz, G. (1978) *FEBS Lett.* 85, 165–170
50. Steer, M. L. and Wood, A. (1979) *J. Biol. Chem.* 254, 10791–10797
51. Aktories, K., Schultz, G. and Jakobs, K. H. (1979) *FEBS Lett.* 107, 100–104
52. Aktories, K., Schultz, G. and Jakobs, K. H. (1980) *N. Z. Arch. Pharmacol.* 372, 167–173
53. Sabol, S. L. and Nirenberg, M. (1979) *J. Biol. Chem.* 254, 1913–1920
54. Londos, C. L., Cooper, D. M. F. and Walff, J. (1980) *Proc. Natl Acad. Sci. U.S.A.* 77, 2551–2554
55. Murad, F., Chi, Y. M., Rall, J. W. and Sutherland, E. W. (1962) *J. Biol. Chem.* 237, 1233–1239
56. Jakobs, K. H., Aktories, K. and Schultz, G. (1979) *N. Z. Arch. Pharmacol.* 310, 113–119
57. Blume, A. J., Lichtstein, D. and Boone, G. (1979) *Proc. Natl Acad Sci. U.S.A.* 76, 5626–5630
58. Koski, G. and Klee, W. B. (1981) *Proc. Natl Acad. Sci. U.S.A.* 79, 4185–4189
59. Steer, M. L., Braun, S., Lester, H. A. and Levitzki, A. (submitted)

Are there differences in the β-receptor–adenylate cyclase systems of fragmented membranes and living cells?

Hartmut Porzig

Pharmakologisches Institut der Universität, Friedbühlstr. 49, CH-3010 Bern, Switzerland.

During the last few years experimental data on biochemical and functional properties of the β-adrenoceptor-adenylate cyclase system have accumulated very rapidly. In spite of the successes of biochemical dissection of receptor–cyclase interactions, the functioning of the β-adrenergic system in the intact cell received much less attention.

The amazing stability of β-receptors during cell fractionation has occasionally favoured a 'grind and bind' philosophy which considered receptor binding studies in intact cells a complication that could be avoided without loss of information. However, recent evidence allows one to define more clearly which aspects of β-adrenergic signal transmission require studies in intact cells. I shall consider three groups of problems which belong to this category: (1) Evaluation of the *in vivo* stoichiometric coupling between receptor occupation and adenylate cyclase activation. (2) Adaptive changes in β-adrenoceptor properties or adenylate cyclase activity upon sustained adrenergic stimulation. (3) Interactions between cell metabolism or other cytosolic factors and adrenergic receptor function.

I shall restrict myself to a discussion of differences in the β-receptor–cyclase system of intact cells and membrane particles (see Table I). However, it is important to point out that the demonstration of *in vivo* receptor–cyclase coupling is not sufficient to identify a given β-adrenergic binding site as the receptor mediating a physiological β-adrenergic response like chronotropic effects in the heart. Such identification is only possible by comparing carefully the properties of specific ligands at the receptor site in intact cells to their properties in eliciting a response distal to cyclase activation.

Methodological problems

The main reason why studies of β-adrenoceptor properties in intact cells were unpopular was the difficulty, at least

TABLE I. Some differences in the β-receptor adenylate cyclase system of intact cells and fragmented membranes

Measured parameter	Intact cells	Membrane particles	Cell system
Desensitization after chronic β-adrenergic stimulation	80–90% decrease in isoprenaline-dependent cAMP formation	35–50% decrease	Human astrocytoma[11]
K_A/K_D ratio for agonists	$\ll 1$	~ 1	rat glioma, S49 lymphoma[5,6]
β-Agonist affinity	Decreased by some antagonists	Not affected by antagonists	Rat heart cells (Porzig, Becker and Reuter, unpublished)
Metabolic dependence of receptor density	Decrease in receptor numbers in starved cells	No effect	Rat reticulocytes[15]
Membrane phospholipid metabolism	β-Adrenergic stimulation in resealed cell ghosts	No effect	Rat reticulocytes[17]
Effect of microtubule disruption agents	Increase in agonist affinity, inhibition of phosphodiesterase induction	–	Polymorphonuclear leucocytes[2] C6 glioma[18]

in most mammalian tissues, of discriminating between stereospecific low capacity binding of β-adrenergic ligands to receptors and nonstereospecific high capacity binding to membranes or intracellular structures. Tissue homogenization usually reduces non-specific binding from 70–80% to 10–20% of total binding. Specific binding is generally defined as that amount of a radiolabelled β-adrenergic antagonist (mostly (−)-[³H]dihydroalprenolol or ¹²⁵I-(±)-hydroxybenzylpindolol (HYP) that can be displaced by a second specific competitive β-receptor ligand. Most adrenergic antagonists, labelled or unlabelled, which are used in such studies have at least two of the following disadvantages. (1) Many are lipophilic, whereas agonists are usually hydrophilic. (2) Some have non-specific, e.g. local anaesthetic, actions on membranes which may cause non-competitive displacement of specific ligands. (3) Some are partial agonists or have affinities to other receptors.

The suppression of non-specific binding sometimes requires intensive washing for prolonged periods of time and addition of the α-adrenergic antagonist phentolamine at high concentrations. These maneuvers could possibly influence β-receptor properties. Consequently the results were open to controversy[1]. Non-specific uptake may in part result from partitioning of ligands into lysosomes, since it is reduced considerably by the lysosomotropic compound chloroquine[2].

In spite of these difficulties, β-receptor properties were measured successfully in a few tissues, especially in cultured cell lines, where non-specific binding is less prominent. Moreover, new β-adrenergic antagonists have been synthesized which do not share some of the disadvantages of the 'pioneer' ligands. Among them are (−)timolol, a pure optical isomer essentially without partial agonistic or local anaesthetic actions, and ¹²⁵I-(±)cyanopindolol, a ligand with high specific activity but, unlike HYP, without affinity for alpha-adrenergic receptors[3]. Finally, (±)-[³H]CGP 12177* is remarkable as a highly hydrophilic β-adrenergic antagonist with high affinity and very little

---
*CGP 12177 was synthesized by Ciba-Geigy and made available to us by Professor M. Staehelin of the Friedrich-Miescher-Institute, Basel, Switzerland.

non-specific binding in living cells (Porzig and Reuter, unpublished results). Fig. 1 shows the binding of [^{3}H]CGP 12177 to intact rat heart cells from a primary tissue culture. The incubation medium for the binding experiment was identical to the normal culture medium. With 1 nM CGP 12177 non-specific binding was less than 10% of total binding.

Receptor–adenylate cyclase coupling

Ever since it became possible to measure specific β-adrenergic binding sites reliably in the mid-1970s, people have tried to establish quantitative correlations between receptor occupancy and the physiological effects of β-adrenergic stimulation. It was soon realized that the apparent affinities of agonists for specific binding sites were often much lower than anticipated from their potencies to elicit a physiological response, e.g. an increase in heart rate. This was to be expected, since these actions involve many reaction steps far away from the drug–receptor interaction. It was somewhat more uncomfortable when it was discovered that in many tissues no direct correlation seemed to exist between receptor occupation by a full agonist and adenylate cyclase activation. The activation of this enzyme is the first measurable step in the sequence following hormone–receptor interaction. A 1:1 coupling between receptor occupancy and enzyme activation would have been the simplest assumption. Later studies revealed that signal transfer from receptor to enzyme required an intermediate guanylnucleotide binding protein (N unit)[4]. Non-linear interactions between these three reactants could, in principle, explain deviations from 1:1 coupling ratios. However, the stoichiometries of these interactions are still unknown because neither the membrane concentrations of N unit and enzyme nor the affinities of both for their respective reaction partners have so far been measured. Therefore, the relation between receptor occupancy and cyclase activity remains the only overall measure for estimating apparent coupling ratios between signal and effect. Before discussing the hypotheses which have been advanced to explain apparent non-linear receptor–effector relationships let us briefly consider their premises.

Many studies have compared quantitatively agonist binding constants (K_D values) in cell homogenates with the agonist concentration required for half maximal stimulation of adenylate cyclase (K_A value). The enzyme was stimulated either in the homogenate or in the intact tissue. Such comparison is based on the implicit assumption that the properties of the receptor–cyclase system in the membrane preparation are identical to those in the intact cell or, at least, that all of its components survive the preparation procedures to the same extent. This assumption is not always justified. In rat reticulocytes the preparation of membranes caused a shift of the K_A but not of the K_D value to higher agonist concentrations. Large differences in K_A/K_D ratios of cells and homogenates

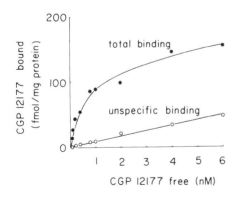

Fig. 1. Equilibrium binding of the β-adrenergic antagonist [^{3}H]CGP 12177 (4-(3-tert-butylamino-2-hydroxypropoxy)-benzimidazol-2-on- [5,7-^{3}H(N)] to living heart cells. K_D value = 0.37 nM. Cell monolayers were incubated in Dulbecco's modified MEM containing 10% fetal calf serum. Specific binding is the difference between total binding and binding in the presence of 10^{-6}M (−)timolol (unpublished results of Porzig, Becker and Reuter).

have been observed in several cultured cell lines[5,6]. In these systems agonists seemed to compete more effectively with antagonists for sites in membranes than for sites in intact cells. What alters the receptor properties in membrane particles as compared to intact cells? K_D values for agonists in cells and membranes are usually calculated from the competitive displacement of a radiolabelled antagonist by increasing agonist concentrations. Estimation of K_D values by this method depends on the assumption that the labelled antagonist does not change receptor properties 'seen' by the agonist. The assumption seems to hold true in membrane preparations. However, in intact cultured rat heart cells we have observed that isoprenaline K_D values were higher by more than an order of magnitude if determined by competitive displacement of the lipophilic antagonist [^{3}H]carazolol ($K_D = 1.6 \times 10^{-6}$M) rather than of the hydrophilic antagonist CGP 12177 ($K_D = 3 \times 10^{-8}$M) (Pörzig, Becker and Reuter, unpublished). Such discrepancies, however, did not exist in crude homogenates obtained from hearts of newborn rats. Moreover, even in intact cells the antagonist timolol was equally potent in displacing the two labelled compounds. Fig. 2 shows that receptor occupation by isoprenaline almost coincides with its stimulatory effect on adenylate cyclase provided the displacement of [^{3}H]CGP 12177 is used to estimate K_D. Analysis of these findings led to the conclusion that several lipophilic antagonists (carazolol, cyanopindolol) are able to lower agonist affinity of β-adrenoceptors in intact cardiac cells. This effect depends on the time of exposure to the antagonists.

In conclusion, misleading results can be obtained if one cannot rely on the inertness of the tools which we use to measure receptor–binding constants. The difference in K_A/K_D ratios between intact cells and isolated membranes is often taken to indicate different degrees of coupling between

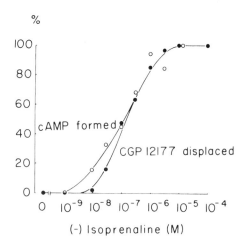

Fig. 2. Correlation between receptor occupancy by isoprenaline and stimulation of cAMP formation in native rat heart cells. The cells were exposed to 5 nM CGP 12177 for 15 min. Isoprenaline was then added and another 15 min later, total accumulation of cAMP or specific displacement of [^{3}H]CGP 12177 was measured. Same incubation medium as in Fig. 1. For the cAMP assay it was supplemented with 1 mM of the phosphodiesterase inhibitor isobutylmethylxanthine. Half maximal effects were reached with 1.3×10^{-7}M isoprenaline in both cases (unpublished results of Pörzig, Becker and Reuter).

receptor and adenylate cyclase[5,6]. However, in most cases the data could be explained equally well by an antagonist-induced decrease in agonist affinity, occurring only in cells, but not in homogenates. A comparison of antagonist K_i and K_D values* in cardiac tissue of different species also suggests an effect of cell homogenization on receptor properties. With some antagonists, K_D values were significantly lower than K_i values[7]. Such differences which are not compatible with the occupancy theory of drug–receptor interaction most probably reflect a homogenization artefact. Nevertheless, real differences in K_A/K_D ratios between tissues seem to exist.

* K_i and K_D symbolize, respectively, the equilibrium dissociation constants for antagonists estimated from inhibition of physiological effects of isoprenaline (e.g. stimulation of cAMP synthesis, positive chronotropic action) or from direct radioligand binding to membrane particles.

Studies with irreversible β-adrenoceptor blocking agents indicate that in some systems occupation of only a small fraction of non-blocked receptors by the agonist can maintain the maximal rate of cyclic AMP accumulation[8].

The various reaction schemes which have been proposed to describe the signal transfer from the receptor to the adenylate cyclase account in two general ways for the deviation from a simple direct proportionality between receptor occupancy and enzyme activity. (1) It is assumed that the number of receptors exceeds by far the number of cyclase molecules ('spare receptor hypothesis'). Consequently, full activation of the enzyme would require only a fraction of the receptors to be occupied by the hormone[9]. (2) Alternatively, and in better agreement with the experimental data, the coupling between the hormone–receptor complex (RH) and adenylate cyclase (C) is assumed to follow a hyperbolic function. Consequently, non-linear functional receptor–effector relationships would result, independently of the stoichiometric relation between receptor and enzyme molecules[4,10]. The coupling function in this context comprises the sum of all intermediary steps between binding of hormone and increase in cyclic AMP. According to this latter concept the observation '$K_A = K_D$' represents a limiting case where the overall affinity (K) of RH for C is small compared to the total receptor concentration ($[R_t]$). On the other hand, '$K_A < K_D$' would result in systems where K is large compared to $[R_t]$.

Intracellular determinants of receptor–adenylate cyclase properties

A large body of evidence has accumulated suggesting that in living cells receptor numbers and binding constants as well as receptor–adenylate cyclase coupling are far from being static properties. Reacting to environmental or internal changes, the cell constantly adjusts its responsiveness to hormonal stimuli. With few exceptions, verification of altered receptor properties has been sought in membrane preparations isolated from *in vivo* treated cells. This method was successful because some of the adaptive changes in the receptor–cyclase system survive the preparation procedure.

Desensitization

In many tissues chronic adrenergic stimulation causes a decrease in hormone-stimulated cyclic AMP synthesis[9]. The detailed mechanism of this phenomenon is still incompletely understood. Only part of it is explained by an apparent loss of β-adrenoceptors which is the most prominent remnant of desensitization in cell homogenates. However, studies on homogenates give only an incomplete picture of the desensitization process in intact cells. In human astrocytoma cells two different processes were shown to account for the 80–90% decrease in the rate of cyclic AMP synthesis upon prolonged β-adrenergic stimulation of intact cells: a hormone-specific ~30% loss of receptors and a hormone non-specific ~50% decrease in cyclase responsiveness caused by factors distal to the receptor[11]. In membrane preparations of these cells the second component of desensitization was completely lost. The authors suggest that some soluble adenylate cyclase inhibitor might have accumulated in the cell during desensitization. It is equally possible that in desensitized cells the coupling function between receptors and cyclase has been altered by some metabolic reaction which is not preserved in membrane preparations.

In a fibroblast cell line from rat kidneys, desensitization of the β-adrenergic stimulation of adenylate cyclase could be demonstrated in a cell-free system[12]. The process required GTP, ATP and Mg^{2+}. The ATP requirement perhaps indicates that desensitization is promoted by an energy-dependent reaction. Nevertheless, it is quite obvious from these studies that neither the time course nor the final extent of cellular desensitization could be modelled exactly in the membrane preparation. Apparently desensitization in living cells is governed by additional factors which are not under control in this system. Two surprising mechanisms have been detected which may contribute to cell-bound desensitization. In brain slices desensitization was rapidly reversed upon tissue depolarization suggesting that membrane voltage can have a regulatory effect on the β-receptor adenylate cyclase system[13].

During desensitization of frog erythrocytes, β-adrenergic binding sites are removed from the membrane surface and transferred into the cytosol by an ATP-dependent endocytotic process[14].

Cellular metabolic activity and receptor properties

ATP depletion by metabolic inhibition of native rat reticulocytes is associated with a ~30% loss of β-receptors and an increase in the affinity of the remaining receptors for agonists[15]. This increase in agonist affinity is probably due to the decrease in intracellular GTP concentration in starved cells. The sensitivity of β-receptors to guanylnucleotides is well preserved during cell homogenization and has been studied extensively[4,16]. Most hypotheses propose that the cyclic association of the guanylnucleotide binding protein (N unit) with either GTP or GDP induces the receptor-N unit complex to assume alternating states of low and high affinities for agonists, respectively. In membrane preparations, saturating concentrations of GTP may drive all receptors into the low affinity state. In the absence of GTP a large fraction of receptors assumes a high affinity state. In living cells the steady state distribution of GTP-dependent receptor affinity states is largely unknown. In native, well-fed rat reticulocytes, a small fraction of high affinity sites always coexists with the low affinity forms, even though the cells contain saturating GTP concentrations and little GDP.

In membranes and in intact cells, GTP is without any effect on receptor densities. How can we explain the loss of receptors which is induced by metabolic inhibition if it is not a GTP-dependent process? An interesting possibility is suggested by studies showing close correlations between membrane lipid metabolism and apparent β-receptor numbers[17]. Stimulation of phospholipid methylation increased the number of β-adrenoceptors in resealed rat reticulocyte ghosts, but not in fragmented membranes. Apparently the treatment exposed preformed, but previously inaccessible, receptors. It did not seem to induce *de novo* receptor synthesis. Formation and incorporation of specific lipids in membranes may be one of the ways by which cells maintain a steady state β-receptor density. A loss of receptors in starved cells would be a logical consequence of this mechanism.

Cytoskeleton and β-adrenergic signal transmission

The presence of microtubules in most intact cells and their disruption during membrane preparation is probably an additional reason for discrepant observations on the β-adrenergic system in living tissue, and in cell homogenates. The microtubule-disrupting agent, colchicine, enhances the potency of isoprenaline to stimulate adenylate cyclase activity. Recent studies on the effect of colchicine in living leukocytes have shown a several-fold increase in β-receptor affinity for the agonist, but no effect on receptor density[2]. The mechanism of this effect is unknown. Possibly microtubules regulate the mobility of receptor proteins within the membrane and hence, may interfere with receptor-N unit or cyclase interactions. Other authors[18] have suggested that the adaptive activation of phosphodiesterase after persistent β-adrenergic stimulation of intact

C6 glioma cells requires intact microtubules. This conclusion was based on the inhibition of this process by vinblastine.

Conclusions

Very detailed knowledge of the principal biochemical properties and the interaction between β-receptors and adenylate cyclase has been obtained from work on isolated membrane particles. Yet, properties and regulation of this system as a mediator of the physiological effects of catecholamines, have to be studied in intact cells. Quite a number of observations indicate that binding constants and cyclase activation characteristics defined in membrane particles cannot be strictly applied to calculate stoichiometric stimulus–effect relationships in living tissues. Some regulatory changes in the β-receptor/adenylate cyclase system, e.g. adaptive increase or decrease in receptor numbers, remain stable during homogenization and membrane preparation. Only intact cell studies will help to decide whether these changes are also physiologically the most important ones.

Reading list

1. Pochet, R. and Schmitt, H. (1979) *Nature (London)* 277, 58–59; reply by Atlas, D., Hanski, E. and Levitzki, A. (1979) *Nautre (London)* 277, 59–60
2. Dulis, B. H. and Wilson, I. B. (1980) *J. Biol. Chem.* 255, 1043–1048
3. Engel, G., Hoyer, D., Berthod, R. and Wagner, H. (1980) *Naunyn-Schmiedebergs Arch. Pharmakol.* 311, R 60
4. Rodbell, M. (1980) *Nature (London)* 284, 17–22
5. Terasaki, W. L. and Brooker, G. (1978) *J. Biol. Chem.* 253, 5418–5425
6. Insel, P. and Stoolman, L. M. (1978) *Mol. Pharmacol.* 14, 549–561
7. Kaumann, A. J., McInerny, T. K., Gilmour, D. P. and Blinks, J. R. (1980) *Naunyn-Schmiedebergs Arch. Pharmakol.* 311, 219–236
8. Terasaki, W. L., Linden, J. and Brooker, G. (1979) *Proc. Natl Acad. Sci. U.S.A.* 76, 6401–6405
9. Williams, L. T. and Lefkowitz, R. J. (1978) *Receptor Binding Studies in Adrenergic Pharmacology*, Raven Press, New York
10. Homburger, V., Lucas, M., Cantau, B., Barabe, J., Pevit, J. and Bockaert, J. (1980) *J. Biol. Chem.* 255, 10436–10444
11. Johnson, G. L., Wolfe, B. B., Harden, T. K., Molinoff, P. B. and Perkins, J. P. (1978) *J. Biol. Chem.* 253, 1472–1480
12. Anderson, W. B. and Jaworski, C. J. (1979) *J. Biol. Chem.* 254, 4596–4601
13. Wagner, H. R. and Davis, J. N. (1979) *Proc. Natl Acad. Sci. U.S.A.* 76, 2057–2061
14. Chuang, D. M., Kinnier, W. J., Farber, L. and Costa, E. (1980) *Mol. Pharmacol.* 18, 348–355
15. Baer, M. and Porzig, H. (1980) *FEBS Lett.* 111, 205–208
16. Ross, E. M. and Gilman A. G. (1980) *Annu. Rev. Biochem.* 49, 533–564
17. Hirata, F. and Axelrod, J. (1980) *Science*, 209, 1082–1090
18. Schwartz, J. P. and Costa, E. (1980) *J. Pharmacol. Exp. Ther.* 212, 569–572

Biochemical and immunochemical analysis of β-adrenergic receptor adenylate cyclase complexes

A. Donny Strosberg, P. O. Couraud, O. Durieu-Trautmann and C. Delavier-Klutchko

Molecular Immunology Laboratory, I.R.B.M. – C.N.R.S. and University of Paris VII, Place Jussieu 2 – 75251 Paris Cedex 05, France

Catecholamine hormone stimulation of adenylate cyclase activity can now be interpreted in molecular terms: binding to a β-adrenergic receptor is followed by GTP-mediated transmission of a signal to the cyclase catalytic unit. Further characterization of the molecules intervening in the various steps is reviewed here. New immunological approaches to analyse the whole system are also discussed.

Recent years have seen an exponential growth of reports concerning the biochemical analysis of hormone and neurotransmitter receptor–effector systems[1]. The studies of the various subunits of the acetylcholine receptor have reached the decisive stage of amino acid sequence determinations as well as morphological characterization by electron microscopy[2]. Progress has not been so rapid for the β-adrenergic receptor cyclase system, mainly because of the lack of tissue equivalent to the electric organ of the Torpedo fish, which contains up to 100,000 receptor molecules per square micron. In their search for a favorable cell, specialists of the β-adrenergic receptors have screened animals as diverse as the frog, turkey, mouse and man, and have studied established cell lines as well as freshly recovered tissues.

Despite these difficulties, the analysis of the catecholamine–sensitive adenylate cyclase systems has continued to attract enormous attention mainly because of the crucial role of catecholamines in human physiology attested by the availability of a large variety of agonist and antagonist compounds. An equally important reason for the interest in the β-adrenergic complex is the opportunity to study in the same system an external hormonal signal and the transmission to the inside of the cell through activation of adenylate cyclase[3–5].

In this review we will summarize the latest developments in the characterization and purification of the various components of the β-adrenergic receptor–cyclase system and will present the features of the system for which a consensus has been reached by the major investigators in the field.

The β-adrenergic receptor

A number of groups now generally agree to the existence in the membranes of a variety of cells of at least one class of high affinity non co-operative catecholamine receptor sites. These molecules remain present on the purified membranes, and have been solubilized with preservation of their pharmacological binding properties.

We will first summarize our present knowledge about the β-adrenergic receptor–adenylate cyclase complex in terms of the functional role of the various components and then review the recent advances in the purification of these constituents by biochemical and immunochemical methods.

Present knowledge of the β-adrenergic system

Adenylate cyclase (C) can be stimulated to increase cAMP production by β-adrenergic catecholamine agonists in a variety of tissues. The order of potency of stimulation by a number of compounds defines the β_1 (isoproterenol > norepinephrine $\geqslant$ epinephrine) or β_2 (isoproterenol > epinephrine > norepinephrine) character of the hormone binding site, the receptor (R). Stimulation of the cyclase catalytic unit, as well as binding to the receptor, is effectively blocked by antagonists such as alprenolol or propranolol. The latter β-blocker is of considerable therapeutic value.

The affinity of the β-adrenergic receptor for agonists is modulated by a GTP binding protein, the G/F regulatory protein, which confers upon cyclase the ability to use its physiological substrate MgATP and the capacity to be activated by fluoride and guanine nucleotides[3–5]. In avian erythrocytes a catecholamine hormone-sensitive

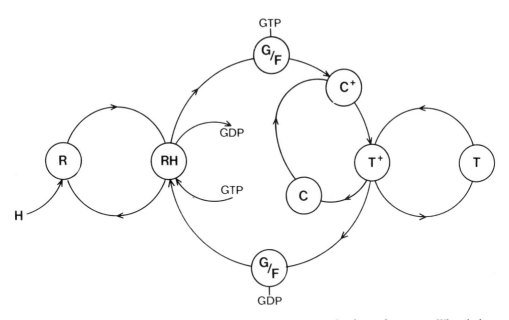

Fig. 1. Catecholamine hormone stimulation of the β-adrenergic receptor–adenylate cyclase system. When the hormone (H), or antibody, specifically binds to the receptor (R), the RH complex acquires a high affinity towards the GDP-bound regulatory protein (G/F). The formation of this ternary complex promotes the replacement of GDP by GTP on the G/F nucleotide binding site, which in turn destabilizes the complex, leading to a free receptor (R) and to an active GTP-bound regulatory protein. This GTP-bound G/F unit now interacts and stimulates the adenylate cyclase (C), leading to the active form C^+. The GTPase unit (T) is stimulated by the GTP-bound G/F protein and hydrolyses the GTP molecule, effecting the turn-off of the response to the hormone signal: the (G/F –C^+) complex is dissociated, the catalytic unit returns to its resting state (C), while the GDP-bound G/F protein is once more ready to associate with RH complex.

GTPase (T) also regulates the stimulation of C by the agonists and GTP: activation of cyclase is short-lived in the presence of GTP and permanent with the non-hydrolysable analog guanyl-5′-yl-imidodiphosphate [Gpp(NH)p][6,7].

A number of models have been presented which attempt to integrate the known interactions between the various components of the β-adrenergic system[4,5]. A consensus, summarized in Fig. 1, could probably be reached on the following features: four functional units, R, G/F, T and C, interact through sequential 'cycling' steps. First the hormone specifically modifies the receptor's conformation causing physical coupling to the G/F protein and activation of a hormone-sensitive GTPase activity. Then, in the presence of GTP, the activated G/F regulatory unit stimulates adenylate cyclase activity. Finally, the hormone-sensitive GTPase, by hydrolysing GTP, returns the system to its resting state.

Two features of this model are striking: (a) the hormone acts only as a trigger for the receptor; in fact other specific ligands, such as anti-receptor antibodies, can play the same role both in terms of binding and in leading to adenylate cyclase activation[8,9]; (b) the triggered receptor itself activates the G/F regulatory protein and GTPase before returning to a less active role. Thus, in fact, the specific components of any hormone-sensitive adenylate cyclase system only intervene in the initial stages of the stimulation or, for that matter, inhibition of catalysis: the same nucleotide regulatory, GTPase and cyclase catalytic units can probably be used in association with various hormone receptors in the same or in different cells. Glucagon, secretin and catecholamines may all use different receptors but the same effector system. More strikingly, the same catecholamines may, by acting through α-receptors instead of through β-receptors, trigger the stimulation of GTPase and inhibition of adenylate cyclase activity[10].

Purification of the β-adrenergic receptor

Advances in the purification of the β-adrenergic receptor have been helped considerably by the availability of radioactive catecholamine hormone agonists and antagonists labeled to very high specific activities. Progress towards the purification has come through the use of affinity chromatography either alone or in combination with immunological methods.

Affinity chromatography of the β-adrenergic receptor was based on the chemical coupling of a potent hormone antagonist to a spacer arm itself attached to a Sepharose inert support[11,12]. Although apparently straightforward, the development of a suitable affinity gel required considerable efforts before a receptor purification factor of about 22,000 could be attained in a single step, starting out from turkey erythrocyte plasma membrane which was solubilized by digitonin[13]. Similar degrees of purification of the frog erythrocyte receptor were reached through three successive affinity chromatographies combined with ion exchange chromatography[14].

TABLE I. Characterization of components from the β-adrenergic receptor from turkey erythrocyte membranes

Study 1 Affinity chromatography	Study 2 Affinity chromatography	Study 3 Immunoprecipitation	Study 4 Immunoprecipitation	Study 5 Affinity labeling
30	26–30			38
33				41
60	58	60	68	
(72)				

The purified frog receptor preparations bind alprenolol with a specific activity of 8–10,000 pmol mg^{-1} of protein, representing a 55,000-fold purification. Sodium dodecyl sulfate-polyacrylamide gel electrophoresis of affinity purified iodinated receptor reveal bands of proteins of 30, 33 and 60 kD for the turkey, and 26–30 and 58 kD for the frog polypeptide chains (Table I).

Various observations from both laboratories suggest that the 58–60 kD component consistently corresponds to the polypeptide chain which contains the hormone binding site, while the 26–33 kD components may actually correspond either to proteolytic fragments of the larger subunit, or to proteins with other functions which copurify on the affinity column and are part of the β-adrenergic receptor–G/F regulatory protein–adenylate cyclase complex. In addition we have most recently been able to detect an additional 72 kD component which was resolved through a two dimensional gel electrophoresis (isoelectric focusing in one direction, SDS electrophoresis in the second dimension) of receptor. This result is presented in Fig. 2.

The G/F regulatory protein and the catecholamine sensitive GTPase

The chromatographically purified G/F, enriched 2000-fold from extracts of rabbit liver plasma membranes reconstitutes guanine nucleotide-, fluoride- and hormone-stimulated adenylate cyclase activity in a variant of S49 murine lymphoma cells deficient in G/F regulatory activity[15]. The purified factor also reconstitutes hormonal stimulation of another variant of these cells. The preparation of enriched G/F contains three polypeptide chains with approximate mol. wts of 35, 45 and 52 K and the active fraction behaves as a multi-subunit complex of these polypeptides which all appear necessary for full function. Treatment of G/F with cholera toxin in the presence of radiolabeled

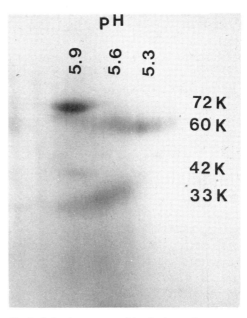

Fig. 2. Subunit structure of the β-adrenergic receptor. Affinity purified receptor was radio-iodinated and submitted to isoelectric focusing using a 3–10 pH gradient and then electrophoresed in the second dimension in SDS. Three major bands are apparent: the 60 K and the 30–33 K bands were previously described[13]; the 72 K band appeared in recent preparations.

NAD$^+$ results in the ADP radioribosylation of the 45 and 52 K polypeptides. No GTPase activity was detected in the purified G/F fraction. None of the components, whether separated or reassembled, display any catecholamine hormone binding.

Whether the GTP binding protein and the catecholamine-sensitive GTPase constitute a single component of the β-adrenergic receptor–cyclase complex or whether they represent different entities is still actively discussed. Four recent series of experiments illustrate the relationship between the GTP regulatory protein, the hormone sensitive GTPase and the β-adrenergic receptor:

1. Cholera toxin inhibits the catecholamine-stimulated GTPase activity in turkey erythrocyte membranes[7,16].

2. NEM inactivates the catecholamine-sensitive GTPase but does not, by itself, affect the receptor. The simultaneous pres-

ence of NEM and catecholamine agonists inactivates about half of the total number of receptors and this inactivation is prevented by GTP or Gpp(NH)p[17]. It is thus likely that the NEM-sensitive site on the receptor is involved in the interaction between the receptor and the GTP regulatory protein.

3. Pretreatment of receptor-containing membranes with agonists plus GMP[18], or plus magnesium and EDTA[19] apparently increases the agonist binding affinity of the receptor. Pretreatment with GMP plus agonist leads to the solubilization by digitonin of the GTPase which remains sensitive to the presence of the catecholamine hormone thus suggesting the preservation of an effective relationship between receptor and GTPase in the soluble extract[20].

4. Using two soluble membrane fractions, one containing the β-adrenergic receptor and the other a GTP binding protein, Citri and Schramm showed that they could recouple these two functional units in a phospholipid environment and then implant the (receptor + GTP binding protein) complex into plasma membranes containing hormone-insensitive adenylate cyclase and obtain hormonal stimulation of the enzyme[21]. If such a reconstitution experiment could be repeated by using purified components, obviously one would have demonstrated that hormonal stimulation of the cyclase catalytic unit requires both the receptor for binding and the GTP binding protein for the transmission. Control experiments with either the receptor or the GTP binding protein-containing fractions only did not lead to cyclase stimulation. Whether additional components are needed thus remains an open question.

Immunological studies of the β-adrenergic receptor–cyclase complex

The previous paragraphs have clearly shown the intricate relationships between the various components of the β-adrenergic receptor–cyclase complex. The receptor which can bind both agonists and antagonists is influenced by the presence of guanine nucleotides as well as by magnesium, and modulates both the activity of a GTPase and of adenylate cyclase, through the interaction with a GTP binding regulatory protein.

The effect of reagents such as DTT or NEM may yield important information concerning the structure of these proteins[22,17]. An essential point in the study of the system, however, concerns the transmission of the hormonal signal through the plasma membrane to the inside of the cell.

To study phenomena such as a receptor redistribution or interaction with proteins of the cellular cytoskeleton, additional tools were clearly needed, and therefore antibodies were prepared that would recognize various elements of the system.

Preparation of anti-receptor antibodies

Anti-turkey erythrocyte receptor antibodies were raised in mice by repeated immunization with the minute amounts of material obtained by specific affinity chromatography. The resulting antibodies were able to hemagglutinate turkey erythrocytes, from which the receptors were initially purified. Other receptor-bearing cells were also recognized, whereas receptor-negative cells were not. Although these antibodies only partially inhibit the binding of β-adrenergic ligands on intact cells, they were shown to recognize the receptor specifically: they immunoprecipitated radiolabeled receptor, they bound receptor–hormone complexes and finally they stained, by immunofluorescence, S49 lymphoma cells known to bear receptors, but not receptor-deficient mutant cells derived from the same line. The anti-receptor antibodies also were shown to stimulate the turkey erythrocyte adenylate cyclase enzyme[8] in the absence and also in the presence of the hormone. A crucial point in these immunological studies concerns the precise step at which the antibodies interact with the β-adrenergic system: do the antibodies interact directly with the receptor? If they do, it must be at a point sufficiently removed from the hormone binding site not to interfere with hormone receptor binding. Do antibodies recognize the GTP regulatory protein? This might explain the basal and the hormone stimulated adenylate cyclase activation.

In fact, these various questions are difficult to answer as long as one works with small amounts of heterogeneous antibodies. A new and exciting technology has now been applied to solve this problem. Homogeneous monoclonal antibodies to the receptor were prepared by fusion between a myeloma-derived vector cell and splenocytes from mice immunized with partially purified receptor preparations from either turkey erythrocytes or calf lung tissue[23]. Whereas we showed that the polyclonal antibodies immunoprecipitate the 60 kD component from the affinity purified turkey erythrocyte receptor, a monoclonal antibody coupled to agarose was shown to retain 22, 31 and 70 kD components from similar receptor preparations[23]. However, only the 70 kD component was eluted by the catecholamine antagonist propranolol.

We have summarized in Table I the different polypeptide chains identified in var-

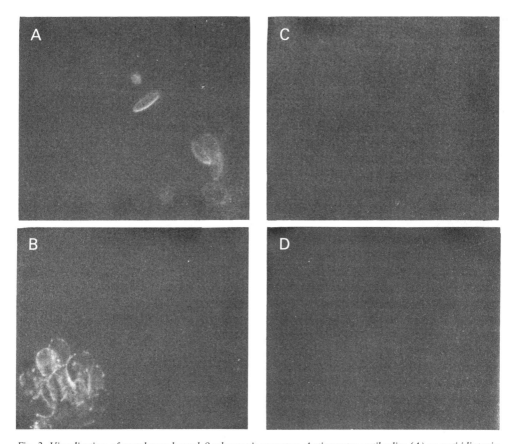

Fig. 3. Visualization of membrane-bound β-adrenergic receptor. Antireceptor antibodies (A) or anti-idiotypic antibodies (B) were absorbed on turkey erythrocytes. Heterologous fluorescent antibodies were used to visualize the membrane-bound binding sites. Similar patterns are observed for the two types of antibodies. Controls with either non-immune sera or cells devoid of β-adrenergic receptor were negative (C, D).

ious β-adrenergic receptor preparations. The convergence of results from very different origins is striking and clearly suggests the progress in this difficult field.

Preparation of anti-anti-hormone antibodies

An alternative immunological approach was suggested by the availability of antibodies raised against β-adrenergic antagonists which also appeared to bind agonists[24]. A report in the literature had indicated that antibodies raised against the active site of anti-insulin antibodies could mimic some of the physiological effects of insulin on adipocytes[25]. This possibility was tested in a system which presented the additional advantage of providing a direct and sensitive way to analyse the hormonal signal, the activation of adenylate cyclase.

The anti-alprenolol antibodies initially obtained in rabbits were purified from the serum and were reinjected in animals with the same genetic background. Anti-antibodies soon appeared in the serum. These were tested for their ability to interact in various ways with the β-adrenergic receptor–cyclase complex. The anti-idiotype antibodies inhibited the binding of hormone on either the antihormone antibody or the membrane-bound receptor[9]. The specific recognition of a turkey erythrocyte plasma membrane protein by the rabbit immunoglobulins could be demonstrated by various methods including binding experiments of radiolabeled antibodies. Control experiments confirmed that β_1 or β_2 receptor-bearing cells from other sources, such as the human HeLa cells, were also recognized whereas receptor negative cells were not. More strikingly, this binding appeared to cause adenylate cyclase stimulation in the absence of hormone[9]. In its presence, increased stimulation was observed. The anti-anti-alprenolol antibodies thus appear to mimic catecholamine hormones both in terms of binding to the receptor and in terms of activation of the adenylate cyclase catalytic unit although the noncompetitivity in binding and synergism in activation clearly suggest differences in the interaction with the adrenergic system.

The anti-idiotypic antibodies do not only serve as useful tools for the functional analysis of the β-adrenergic system: they can actually serve to immunoprecipitate the 60 kD subunit of the β-receptor. In fact, from all points of view, the anti-idiotype antibodies behave in a very similar fashion to the antibodies raised against the purified receptor itself: this is best visualized in the immunofluorescence photographs in Fig. 3A and B.

Conclusion

A comparison of the data reviewed here and those discussed by us only 2 years ago[26], dramatizes the important progress achieved towards the biochemical and now immunochemical characterization of the β-adrenergic receptor–cyclase complex. Whereas affinity chromatography has indeed kept its promise to yield a purified receptor, the application of immunological tools will undoubtedly be of considerable advantage for further functional and structural analysis of the various polypeptide chains which compose the hormone-sensitive system. The exquisite specificity of hybridoma produced monoclonal antibodies and the amazing potential of anti-hormone anti-idiotypic antibodies, which allow us to bypass the preparation of purified receptor, have only been explored very recently[27].

Last but not least, the anti-receptor antibodies will constitute the necessary link between the receptor pharmaco-biochemists and the molecular biologists. *In vitro* translation products of putative receptor coding genes will certainly be analysed immunochemically.

Acknowledgements

We are very grateful to A. Schmutz for

his expert technical assistance, and to J. Hoebeke and E. Strosberg for helpful comments. This work was supported by C.N.R.S., D.G.R.S.T. (No. 79.7.054 and 79.7.0780), I.N.S.E.R.M. (No. 80.1017), Solvay-Tournay, I.W.O.N.L./Janssen Pharmaceutica and F.G.W.O.

Reading list

1 Lamble, J. W. (ed.) (1981) *Towards Understanding Receptors*, Elsevier/North-Holland
2 Giraudat, J. and Changeux, J. P. (1981) *Towards Understanding Receptors* (Lamble, J. W., ed.), pp. 34–43, Elsevier/North-Holland
3 Ross, E. M. and Gilman, A. G. (1980) *Annu. Rev. Biochem.* 49, 533–564
4 Lefkowitz, R. J. and Hoffman, B. B. (1980) *Trends Pharmacol. Sci.* 1, 314–318
5 Rodbell, M. (1980) *Nature (London)* 284, 17–22
6 Cassel, D. and Selinger, Z. (1976) *Biochim. Biophys. Acta* 452, 538–551
7 Cassel, D. and Selinger, Z. (1977) *Proc. Natl Acad. Sci. U.S.A.* 74, 3307–3311
8 Couraud, P. O., Delavier-Klutchko, C., Durieu-Trautmann, O. and Strosberg, A. D. (1981) *Biochem. Biophys. Res. Commun.* 99, 1295–1302
9 Schreiber, A. B., Couraud, P. O., André, C., Vray, B. and Strosberg, A. D. (1980) *Proc. Natl Acad. Sci.* 77, 7385–7389
10 Aktories, K. and Jakobs, K. H. (1981) *FEBS Lett.* 130, 235–238
11 Vauquelin, G., Geynet, P., Hanoune, J. and Strosberg, A. D. (1977) *Proc. Natl Acad. Sci. U.S.A.* 74, 3710–3714
12 Vauquelin, G., Geynet, P., Hanoune, J. and Strosberg, A. D. (1979) *Eur. J. Biochem.* 98, 543–556
13 Durieu-Trautmann, O., Delavier-Klutchko, C., André, C., Vauquelin, G. and Strosberg, A. D. (1980) *J. Supramol. Struct.* 13, 411–419
14 Schorr, R. G. L., Lefkowitz, R. J. and Caron, M. G. (1981) *J. Biol. Chem.* 256, 5820–5826
15 Northup, J. K., Sternweis, P. C., Smigel, M. D., Schleifer, L. S., Ron, E. M. and Gilman, A. G. (1980) *Proc. Natl Acad. Sci. U.S.A.* 77, 6516–6520
16 Cassel, D. and Pfeuffer, T. (1978) *Proc. Natl Acad. Sci. U.S.A.* 77, 2669–2673
17 Vauquelin, G., Bottari, S., André, C., Jacobson, B. and Strosberg, A. D. (1980) *Proc. Natl Acad. Sci. U.S.A.* 77, 3801–3805
18 Lad, P. M., Nielsen, T. B., Preston, M. S. and Rodbell, M. (1980) *J. Biol. Chem.* 255, 988–995
19 Caron, M. G., Limbird, L. E. and Lefkowitz, R. J. (1979) *Mol. Cell Biochem.* 28, 45–66
20 Delavier-Klutchko, C., Durieu-Trautmann, O., Couraud, P. O., André, C. and Strosberg, A. D. (1980) *FEBS Lett.* 117, 341–343
21 Citri, Y. and Schramm, M. (1980) *Nature (London)* 287, 297–300
22 Vauquelin, G., Bottari, S., Kanarek, L. and Strosberg, A. D. (1979) *J. Biol. Chem.* 254, 4462–4469
23 Fraser, C. M. and Venter, J. C. (1980) *Proc. Natl Acad. Sci. U.S.A.* 77, 7034–7038
24 Hoebeke, J., Vauquelin, G. and Strosberg, A. D. (1978) *Biochem. Pharmacol.* 27, 1527–1532
25 Sege, K. and Peterson, P. A. (1978) *Proc. Natl Acad. Sci. U.S.A.* 75, 2443–2447
26 Strosberg, A. D., Vauquelin, G., Durieu-Trautmann, O., Delavier-Klutchko, C., Bottari, S. and André, C. (1980) *Trends Biochem. Sci.* 5, 11–14
27 Strosberg, A. D., Couraud, P. O. and Schreiber, A. B. (1981) *Immunol. Today* 2, 75–79

Immunological studies of hormone receptors: a two-way approach

A. Donny Strosberg, P.-Olivier Couraud and Alain Schreiber

Molecular Immunology Laboratory, I.R.B.M. – C.N.R.S. and University of Paris VII, Place Jussieu 2 – 75251 Paris Cedex 05, France

Recent progress in hormone–receptor studies has resulted from a multidisciplinary approach involving pharmacologists, endocrinologists and biochemists. Immunology provides both tools and a source of concepts for these studies. Endocrine and immune networks share important features which become recognized both by the analysis of autoimmune diseases and of conventionally induced immune responses. The latest discoveries are discussed here.

The recent availability of radiolabeled hormone agonists and antagonists has increased our knowledge about cell surface hormone receptors considerably. After a long period of pharmacological studies, hormone-binding sites obtained from solubilized plasma membranes have been shown to constitute a single class of high affinity receptors with typical protein properties.

Hormone action however, is not only dependent on binding to these receptors; transmission of the signal to the membrane and the interior of the cell clearly requires the presence of one or several additional components which play regulatory and effector functions.

The isolation of the various components, the study of their interaction in the membrane or in solution and their reconstitution into a fully hormone-responsive system still constitute goals which are unlikely to be reached in the very near future. Elegant short cuts obtained by fusing cells which have been genetically or chemically deprived of hormone-responsive complexes have permitted us to assign respective roles to various elements of the systems.

The complexity of the interactions in the endocrine network as well as the specificity of the hormone-responsive components have prompted new experiments involving the immune response against the hormone and its specific receptor. In addition, a number of diseases have been identified in which auto-immune responses interfere with the normal physiological effects of hormones. Some of the salient features of both Nature's and the immunologists' experiments are discussed here.

Hormone–receptor and hormone–antibody interactions

Immunologists have known for a long time that Nature has a variety of solutions to the problem of fitting antibody-combining sites around a given ligand. The fit may be loose or strenuous, the antigen-specific cavity tailored exactly to the size of the determinant, or much larger

Less is known about the hormone binding site on the receptor. In certain systems, a large number of structural or functional hormone analogs may interact with a specific receptor; a variety of catecholamine agonists will bind to the same membrane sites, to either stimulate adenylate cyclase or regulate calcium fluxes. In addition, the same hormones may interact with distinct receptors; thus, acetylcholine will bind both nicotinic and muscarinic receptors and adrenaline will bind both alpha and beta receptors. Whether these different receptors share constant structural features is not known at the present time.

As a rule, the binding constants of receptors for their natural ligands, that is for hormones known to be available in the same organism, are relatively high when compared to the antibody's affinities. This most probably results from a continuous selection process which, when allowed to proceed during an immune response, also generates higher binding constants for an antigen.

Alternatively, the very low concentration of free hormone, in order to be effective, must be compensated by high affinity for the receptor.

A comparison between receptor and antibody properties should not be limited to the exquisite binding properties of the discriminator part of the molecule; the 'second messenger' model of Sutherland included in the receptor complex both transducer and effector components for which the present day equivalents are the guanine nucleotide (GTP) binding regulatory protein and the GTPase and adenylate cyclase catalytic units.

Antibodies can similarly be resolved in antigen-binding regions (V) and effector parts (CH_2/CH_3) which trigger Fc receptors or complement components. A comparison of two independently drawn models (Fig. 1) clearly outlines the similarities between the two molecular recognition complexes. Both are characterized by dual functions; extremely specific recognition by the antigen or hormone binding part

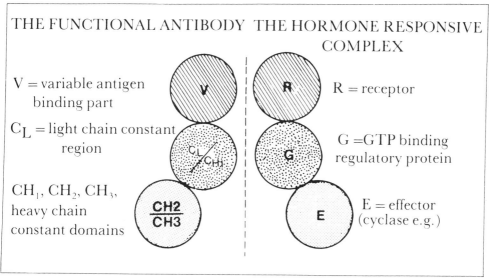

Fig. 1. Conceptual homologies between the antibody molecule and the hormone receptor. Both types of multifunctional structures comprise a recognition moiety (R or V) capable of binding specifically either the antigen or the hormone, a component responsible for signal transmission (C or G) and an effector part (CH2, CH3 or E) responsible for the biological response induced by antigen binding (such as complement fixation or interaction with Fc receptors) or by hormone binding (adenylate cyclase activation, opening of ion channels or phosphorylation).

and activation, through this binding, of well conserved biological effector functions.

Such a juxtaposition raises the question of the existence of a constant part of the receptor–effector complex, a question difficult to answer as long as molecular characterizations are unavailable. The fact that a GTP binding protein regulates the activity of many hormone–receptor complexes and that separate receptors may interact with the same adenylate cyclase suggest a common, constant pathway for different hormones; observations made concerning polypeptide hormones acting through protein kinases and phosphorylations are similar. These findings, as well as many other pharmacological observations, have convinced endocrinologists that a clear image of the structure of hormone receptors will only emerge from a thorough analytical approach involving qualitative and quantitative studies of the binding of the hormone and its agonistic or antagonistic analogs followed by the isolation of the various components of the receptor–cyclase complex. From descriptions of the latest studies it will appear to the readers that immunology provides a striking example and a unique tool for the study of the receptors.

Anti-receptor antibodies

Auto-immune diseases

The recent discovery that myasthenia gravis is an auto-immune disease in which auto-antibodies against the nicotinic–acetylcholine receptor play a major role[1,2] has generated a renewed interest for other examples in which pathological developments may result from the induction of antibodies against hormone receptors: in Graves' hyperthyroidism, serum auto-antibodies are found which bind to the thyroid-stimulating hormone receptor[3,4]; anti-insulin receptor antibodies are found in a rare form of diabetes mellitus, the type B syndrome of insulin resistance with acanthosis nigricans[5,6]. The possible role of auto-antibodies directed against $\beta 2$ – adrenergic receptors was also recently discussed in relation to allergic rhinitis and asthma[7].

These various auto-antibodies interact in different ways with the receptor against which they are directed. Antibodies to the acetylcholine receptor may block the biological response to the hormone, the opening of the ion gate, without interfering with the binding of the hormone to the receptor.

In the sera of patients with the type B syndrome of insulin resistance, antibodies inhibit the binding of insulin and mimic the biological response induced by the hormone, that is the stimulation of glucose uptake by adipocytes[6]. Individual variations in the effects of antibodies clearly suggest that a variety of antigenic determinants may be recognized at the surface of the receptor molecule. Most of the auto-antibodies probably remain undetected since their appearance has no clinical consequence.

Antibodies raised by immunization with purified receptors

The recognition that auto-antibodies may play a major role in some forms of human disease prompted scientists to induce similar reactions in animals by immunization with purified hormone receptors. Experimental myasthenia gravis was thus caused in rabbits or mice by the production of antibodies in response to injections of purified acetylcholine receptors obtained from *Electrophorus electricus*[8]. The man-made disease could be transferred to other animals by administration of the isolated antibodies.

As expected, a wide spectrum of antibody specificities was obtained. Some antibodies blocked both the binding and the biological effect of the hormone; this was reported for antiprolactin receptor[2] and anti-cardiac muscle β receptor[10] antibodies. Blocking of the receptor function without inhibition of hormone binding was described for anti-acetylcholine receptor antibodies[11].

More strikingly, two examples were presented in which anti-receptor antibodies did not interfere with hormone binding but mimicked its physiological action; anti-insulin receptor antibodies were shown to stimulate glucose uptake[12] and anti-catecholamine receptor antibodies could activate the β-adrenergic receptor-associated adenylate cyclase[13].

Since the genetic background of immunized animals and the natural heterogeneity of the antibodies probably account for most of these variables, research was carried out to limit this diversity.

Heterogeneity of conventionally raised antibodies: usefulness of monoclonal antibodies

One inherent difficulty of using fortuitously or conventionally raised anti-receptor antibodies as analytical tools resides in their natural heterogeneity. The antibodies may be directed against each of the various antigenic determinants of the receptor used for immunization or they may specifically recognize other parts of the receptor–transducer–effector complex which accidentally induced the auto-immune reaction.

This explains why anti-receptor antibodies only rarely inhibit the binding of specific ligands and why recognition may cause a variety of physiological responses such as inhibition or stimulation of adenylate cyclase activity, ion fluxes, in the absence or the presence of hormones or guanine nucleotides. The heterogeneity of these antibodies does not allow a precise investigation of the role of each antigenic site in the triggering of a physiological response. However, it does provide a wealth of different reagents which, if they were to be separated, would permit comparative studies of the roles of the various components of the hormone–responsive complex.

Such a separation method is now available; antibody-producing cells can be fused with permanently growing myeloma cells[14]. The resulting hybrids ('hybridomas') can be separated physically by cloning and each can be analysed for their capacity to produce 'monospecific' antibodies. Since such a 'monoclonal' reagent is by definition restricted in its recognition range, it allows an extremely precise analysis of the receptor–effector system.

Monoclonal antibodies against the acetylcholine receptor have been raised by several groups[15–18]. In these studies, only a single clone, out of hundreds that were screened, produced monoclonal antibodies directed against the acetylcholine binding site[18]. This rarity obviously reflects the fact that inhibition of binding by antisera directed against purified receptor was never reported. With this difficulty in mind, one should obviously not screen for monoclonal anti-receptor antibodies only by tests of inhibition of ligand binding. Other screening tests are available such as visualization of immunoglobulin binding to receptor-bearing cells or membranes, and co-precipitation by anti-antibodies of hormone–receptor complexes.

Uses of anti-receptor antibodies

Antibodies which bind hormone receptors have already been used in many ways, ranging from purely morphological to exquisitely analytical studies.

Labeled with fluorescent dyes or radioisotopes, such antibodies can be used to localize the receptor molecules in tissues, or more precisely at the surface of cells. In dynamic studies, the redistribution of receptors can be followed under various physiological conditions. In this case, however, antibodies should not merely be considered as purely passive; by mimicking the hormone, antibodies may, through specific binding to the receptor, induce microaggregation, redistribution and possibly futher cellular metabolic changes. Bivalency of anti-insulin-receptor antibodies appears to play a major role in the mimicking of insulin function; monovalent Fab fragments were unable to imitate the hormonal effects[19].

Since the majority of receptor-binding antibodies do not interfere with hormone recognition, simultaneous effects can be studied, and antibodies can be used to isolate hormone–receptor complexes.

Isolation of receptors by antibody-containing affinity-chromatography gels obviously constitutes one of the major uses of specific antibodies. As long as the availability of these reagents depended on the availability of purified receptors, the advantage over the more classical hormone-containing affinity gels was not clear. The availability of unlimited amounts of monoclonal antibodies even after immunization with crude receptor preparations has eliminated the necessity of prior purification. Acetylcholine receptor has been purified by affinity chromatography on monoclonal antibodies[20]. Monoclonal antibodies also allowed the localization of the main immunogenic region of the acetylcholine receptor and detection of similarities between subunits[17].

More familiar uses of anti-receptor antibodies should also be recalled here; specific antibodies raised against hormone binding molecules purified from one species may be used in phylogenetic studies. An immunological comparison at different stages of the development of a single organism may reveal ontogeny-related changes. Finally, structural relationship between functionally different sites which recognize the same hormone or between receptors which bind structurally homologous ligands may be identified by antibodies.

Anti-hormone antibodies
Diversity of anti-hormone antibodies

The production of antibodies directed against hormones, generally coupled to carriers, illustrates yet another interface between pharmacological and immunological approaches. Such antibodies have been raised against a great variety of pharmacologically active drugs and hormones but only recently have attempts been made to compare the physiological receptors with their immunological image, the antibodies.

While we have discussed some of the similarities in our introduction, obvious differences should be borne in mind.

Thus, the variability of the antibody active site, an inherent advantage of the immune system, does not have its endocrine equivalent; when one compares insulins of different species, the binding constants for various antibody populations may be very dissimilar, but they are quite close for insulin receptors of different origins. In addition, preliminary studies of purified receptors with the same pharmacological properties strongly suggest their conservation, not only in different tissues from the same animal species but also in various species.

The diversity of anti-hormone antibodies expresses itself by the fact that some may compete with the receptor for binding to the ligand while others may bind to hormone determinants removed from the part recognized by the receptor. These latter antibodies may be utilized to isolate hormone–receptor complexes, as was done for the insulin receptor[21].

Anti-hormone antibodies as immunological images of the receptor

Anti-hormone antibodies are evidently directed against a variety of structures recognized on the hormone. In the study of the immune response against β-adrenergic ligands, we noted the particular antigenicity of the pharmacologically active ethanolamine side-chain[22]. Thus, antibodies raised against alprenolol, a strong catecholamine antagonist, not only had a higher binding constant for propranolol, another antagonist, but also bound agonists possessing the ethanolamine group[22].

The question may be raised whether the pharmacologically active side-chain displays pro-eminent structural features explaining the immunodominant position.

Anti-hormone antibodies as stimulators of hormone action

Anti-hormone antibodies may even amplify hormone-induced receptor clustering by cross-linking hormone–receptor complexes. Thus, the exposure of cells to subliminal concentrations of insulin or epidermal growth factor (EGF) followed by the addition of anti-insulin or anti-EGF bivalent antibodies respectively enhanced the biological activity of the hormones[23,24].

Competition of binding and enhancement of hormone action may take place simultaneously when conventionally induced anti-hormone antibodies are used. Monoclonal antibodies would allow a precise analysis of the antibody effect.

Anti anti-hormone antibodies: hormone-like anti-idiotypic reagents

Anti-hormone antibodies turned out to constitute invaluable tools for the possible induction of a hormone-like immunological 'internal image'.

The concept of an internal image was initially proposed by Jerne[25] to explain why mammals could invariably produce antibodies against any type of natural or synthetic antigen. The hypothesis states that any immunoglobulin constitutes an antibody and an antigen recognized as such by other antibodies. This Janus-like internal antigen presents homologies with other foreign antigens; the internal image thus induces the production of antibodies which in turn recognize the foreign material.

Antigen, antibodies and anti-antibodies (the 'anti-idiotypic' reagents) would consti-

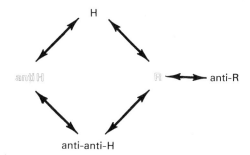

Fig. 2. A network of immunological interactions involving a hormone and its specific receptor. The symmetrical positions of H and anti-anti-H around the receptor have indeed yielded a specific interaction of the anti-anti-H antibodies with R, and receptor, similar in fact to that observed with the anti-R antibody.

tute a network of interactions possibly involving idiotype-bearing T-lymphocytes as well. Endocrine equivalents of such a network may exist: endorphins have been identified as the internal image of the pain-quelling morphine.

By choosing a hormone as the initial antigen, one can verify that the antibody directed against the combining site of the anti-hormone antibody occupies a symmetrical position in regard to the hormone (Fig. 2) since both are recognized by the anti-hormone antibody.

If that is indeed so, would the anti-anti-hormone antibody share other recognition patterns with the hormone? This intriguing question was partially answered by Sege and Peterson who showed that anti-insulin antibodies did bind to insulin receptor-bearing cells and mimicked the insulin-mediated glucose uptake by adipocytes[26].

A more precise analysis of the anti-idiotype antibody hormone-like activity required, however, the investigation of an endocrine system in which not only receptor binding but also hormonal signal transmission and effector activity could be accurately monitored. The catecholamine-stimulated β-adrenergic receptor-adenylate cyclase fulfilled these requirements.

Antibodies against alprenolol, a powerful β-adrenergic antagonist, were raised in rabbits and were shown to be specific for the ethanolamine side-chain present both in catecholamine agonists and antagonists. Anti-idiotypic antibodies did inhibit the binding of the β-adrenergic ligands to these anti-alprenolol antibodies[27]. More striking however, was the fact that the anti-idiotype Ig could also bind to cells and to purified membranes known to display β-receptors on their surface. Appropriate controls were negative.

The transmission of the hormone-binding signal to the cell surface was investigated by studying the activity of the catecholamine-sensitive adenylate cyclase in the presence of the anti-idiotype antibodies. Both the basal and epinephrine-stimulated activities were significantly amplified by the antibodies indicating that the interaction with the receptor can be transmitted to the other components of the β-adrenergic complex.

Both in Sege and Peterson's study and in our own, the antibodies with the hormone-like activity were only synthesized for a short time; their titer rapidly decreased in the serum of the immunized animals. One explanation for this phenomenon was the induction of antibodies of the 'third kind' that is, those directed against the combining site of the anti-idiotype antibodies.

If such antibodies could arise naturally, and not only by intensive immunizations, then one could predict that they would somehow form an active part of the hormone-antibody, hormone-like-antibody network. In a symmetrical arrangement, the anti-anti-idiotypic antibodies would be predicted to bind the hormone, and this is precisely what was found for the catecholamine immunological network; hormone-binding activity appeared concomitantly with the decrease of adenylate cyclase stimulating antibodies (unpublished results).

There is little doubt that the network of immunological interaction involving the β-adrenergic receptor will yield a wealth of useful analytical tools. But it also provides important conceptual interpretations. The hormone-like antibody may actually interfere with the regular endocrine interactions and modify normal physiological patterns with possible pathological consequences.

Conclusions

Immunological studies of hormones and their specific receptors whether in autoimmune diseases or in experimental situations, have provided a wealth of information regarding hormone–receptor interactions.

The ability of anti-receptor antibodies, or anti-anti-hormone antibodies, to mimic hormone action on cells inter-relates endocrine and immunological networks and illustrates the similarities in molecular recognition and effector activation mechanisms.

Once again the fundamental unity in Biology is verified.

Acknowledgements

We are very grateful to J. Hoebeke and E. Strosberg for their helpful assistance. This work was supported by C.N.R.S., D.G.R.S.T. (No. 79.7.054 and 79.7.0780), I.N.S.E.R.M. (No. 80.1017), Solvay-Tournay, I.W.O.N.L./Janssen Pharmaceutika and F.G.W.O. A.S. is a research fellow of N.F.W.O.

Reading list

1 Aharonov, A., Abramsky, O., Tarrab-Hazdai, R. and Fuchs, S. (1975) *Lancet* ii, 340–342
2 Almon, R. R. and Appel, S. H. (1975) *Biochem. Biophys. Acta* 393, 66–77
3 Smith, B. R. and Hall, R. (1974) *Lancet* ii, 427–430
4 Qasim Mehdi, S. and Nussey, S. S. (1975) *Biochem. J.* 145, 105–11
5 Flier, J. S., Kahn, C. R., Roth, J. and Bar, R. S. (1975) *Science* 190, 63–65
6 Kahn, C. R., Baird, K., Flier, J. S. and Jarrett, D. B. (1977) *J. Clin. Invest.* 60, 1094–1106
7 Venter, J. C., Fraser, C. M. and Harrison, L. C. (1980) *Science* 207, 1361–1363
8 Patrick, J., Lindstrom, J., Culp, B. and McMillan,

J. (1973) *Proc. Natl Acad. Sci. U.S.A.* 70, 3334–3338

9 Shiu, R. P. C. and Driesen, H. G. (1976) *Science* 192, 259–261

10 Wrenn, S. and Haber, E. (1978) *J. Biol. Chem.* 254, 6577–6582

11 Lindstrom, J. (1976) *J. Supramol. Struct.* 4, 389–403

12 Jacobs, S., Chang, K. J. and Cuatrecasas, P. (1978) *Science* 200, 1283–1284

13 Couraud, P.-O., Delavier Klutchko, C., Durieu-Trautmann, O. and Strosberg, A. D. (1981) *Biochem. Biophys. Res. Commun.* 99, 1295–1302

14 Kohler, G. and Milstein, C. (1975) *Nature (London)* 256, 495–497

15 Gomez, C. M., Richman, D. P., Berman, P. W., Burres, S. A., Arnason, B. G. W. and Fitch, F. W. (1979) *Biochem. Biophys. Res. Commun.* 88, 575–582

16 Moshly-Rosen, D., Fuchs, S. and Eshhar, Z. (1979) *FEBS Lett.* 106, 389–392

17 Tzartos, S. J. and Lindstrom, J. M. (1980) *Proc. Natl Acad. Sci. U.S.A.* 77, 755–759

18 James, R. W., Kato, A. C., Rey, M. J. and Fulpius, B. W. (1980) *FEBS Lett.* 120, 145–148

19 Kahn, C. R., Baird, K. L., Jarrett, D. B. and Flier, J. S. (1978) *Proc. Natl Acad. Sci. U.S.A.* 75, 4209–4213

20 Lennon, V. A., Thompson, M. and Chen, J. (1980) *J. Biol. Chem.* 255, 4395–4398

21 Heinrich, J., Pilch, P. F. and Czeh, M. P. (1980) *J. Biol. Chem.* 255, 1732–1737

22 Hoebeke, J., Vauquelin, G. and Strosberg, A. D. (1978) *Biochem. Pharmacol.* 27, 1527–1532

23 Schechter, Y., Hernaez, L., Schlessinger, J. and Cuatrecasas, P. (1979) *Nature (London)* 278, 835–838

24 Schlessinger, J. (1980) *Trends Biochem. Sci.* 5, 210–214

25 Jerne, N. K. (1973) *Sci. Am.* 229, 52–60

26 Sege, K. and Peterson, P. A. (1978) *Proc. Natl Acad. Sci. U.S.A.* 75, 2443–2447

27 Schreiber, A. B., Couraud, P. O., Andre, C., Vray, B. and Strosberg, A. D. (1980) *Proc. Natl Acad. Sci. U.S.A.* 77, 7385–7389

Catecholamine-induced modification of the functional state of β-adrenergic receptors

John P. Perkins

Department of Pharmacology, University of North Carolina, Chapel Hill, NC 27514, U.S.A.

Within the plasma membrane of cells there are a variety of proteins involved in the reception, transduction and amplification of extracellular signals. Neurotransmitters and many hormones serve as intercellular signal molecules that alter target cell function upon interaction with cell surface, structure-specific receptors. Beta adrenergic receptors (BAR) can be included in this class of plasma membrane proteins that mediate intercellular communication; it is one aspect of the regulation of this function that is the subject of this article.

The idea that target cell response is a function of the extracellular concentration of the signal molecule is well documented. However, the observation that cells, tissues and animals can exhibit refractoriness (tachyphylaxis) to the effects of administered neurotransmitters, hormones, or their analogs, indicates that variation in the response of a cell to the same concentration of an effector is possible. Similarly, states of 'super responsiveness' can be induced in tissues of animals after surgical or pharmacological manipulation of neural pathways or hormone-secreting organs. Such states of lowered or heightened responsiveness are also observed in certain disease conditions. For example, target tissues for catecholamines exhibit decreased responsiveness in patients with pheochromocytoma, and hyperresponsiveness in patients or in animals with hyperthyroidism. Thus, it seems reasonable to conclude that the capacity of cells to respond to intercellular signals is a dynamic rather than a static process and that such processes must be regulated.

BAR mediate, at least in part, the effects of neurally-released norepinephrine on postsynaptic cells[1]. Of pertinence to this discussion is the observation that when noradrenergic neural activity is chronically increased or decreased the sensitivity to catecholamines of the BAR-linked adenylate cyclase of postsynaptic structures is decreased or increased, respectively[2,3]. The speculation can be put forth that adaptive changes in this enzyme system mediate the associated adaptive changes in the function of postsynaptic systems. Evidence in support of this concept has come from experiments designed to determine if modification of noradrenergic neuronal activity *in vivo* leads to compensatory changes in the BAR-adenylate cyclase system.

Pharmacological perturbation of norepinephrine synthesis, storage and re-uptake has been used as one strategy to change the steady-state level of norepinephrine to which postsynaptic receptors are exposed. For example, central noradrenergic pathways in rats have been destroyed by intraventricular injection of

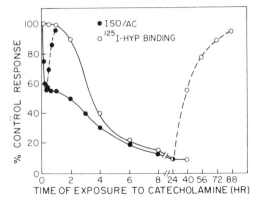

Fig. 1. Time courses of desensitization and reversal of desensitization of isoproterenol-stimulated adenylate cyclase activity and IHYP binding to β-adrenergic receptors. Cells were incubated with 1 μM isoproterenol. At the times indicated, isoproterenol-stimulated adenylate cyclase activity (●) and β-adrenergic receptor density (○) were determined in membrane preparations. The symbols connected by dashed lines indicate the recovery of enzyme activity or β-receptor number after washing the cells free of isoproterenol at the indicated times.

6-hydroxydopamine (6-HDA)[4]. Four days after 6-HDA treatment, a two-fold increase occurred in the maximal accumulation of cyclic AMP inducible by norepinephrine in slices of cerebral cortex. Such results have been interpreted as reflecting postsynaptic adaptation of the adenylate cyclase system in response to the cessation of noradrenergic input. Similarly, reserpine blocks the storage of norepinephrine in nerve endings and thereby reduces noradrenergic neuronal activity. Like 6-HDA, reserpine has been shown to cause hyperresponsiveness to norepinephrine of the cyclic AMP generating system of slices from various areas of the rat brain. Physical denervation studies have generated results that are consonant with the chemical denervation studies utilizing 6-HDA or reserpine. Conversely, when the turnover of norepinephrine was *increased* by chronic administration of amphetamine to mice, slices of cerebral cortex exhibited a submaximal rise in cyclic AMP upon challenge with norepinephrine[5]. Similarly, agents like imipramine, which inhibit re-uptake of neuronally-released norepinephrine, caused a decrease in responsiveness of cortical slices to norepinephrine as well as a loss of BAR as measured by loss of binding sites for the BAR antagonist [^{125}I]iodohydroxybenzylpindolol (IHYP)[6]. Such experimental evidence supports the idea that chronic, excessive noradrenergic nerve activity results in a compensatory decrease in the responsiveness of postsynaptic adenylate cyclase to norepinephrine; whereas, prolonged periods of reduced nerve activity result in an increase in enzyme responsiveness.

Adaptive changes, similar in certain ways to those observed in the intact nervous system, have been observed in non-neuronal cells in culture; in fact, agonist-induced changes in the responsiveness of adenylate cyclase to its effectors appears to be a general response of the enzyme system[2,7,8]. It follows that if the compensatory adaptations of the adenylate cyclase system observed in cultured cells occur as a result of mechanisms similar to those operating in the intact animal, then it might be possible to carry out an examination of the molecular basis of a physiologically important regulatory process in simple model systems.

Studies with catecholamine-responsive cultured cells have been carried out over the past 5–7 years and the results allow the following conclusions. There appear to be at least two basic mechanisms subserving catecholamine-induced desensitization of BAR-linked adenylate cyclase systems. One process is non-specific in nature and has been studied in detail by Brooker, Terasaki and co-workers[7] using the 2B clone of the C6 rat glioma cell line. This process is dependent on protein synthesis and appears to involve a rapidly turning over 'refractoriness' protein. The evidence is mounting that such nonspecific desensitization is mediated by cyclic AMP. Direct binding studies did not indicate any loss of BAR during the first 3 h of the desensitization process in C6-2B cells[7] suggesting that the lesion in the activation process occurs distal to the receptor. This results in a reduction in the capacity of the desensitized enzyme to respond to any of its normal stimulators.

Another mechanism, studied by a number of workers in the field, results in agonist-specific alterations that change only the capacity of the adenylate cyclase system to respond to catecholamines. Based on the current perception of the structure of the catecholamine-specific adenylate cyclase it is reasonable to expect that agonist-specific desensitization would involve a change in the number, or the functional state of the receptor protein specific for the agonist. At least two processes, both involving selective modification of the BAR, appear to account for the agonist-specific component of catecholamine-induced desensitization observed in many cell types.

Su et al.[11] demonstrated that incubation of 132INI astrocytoma cells with isoproterenol results in a rapid ($t_{\frac{1}{2}}$ = 3 min) decrease of catecholamine-stimulated adenylate cyclase activity to a new, essentially steady state level of 40–50% of control. During this time there was no alteration in the number of BAR or in any of the other parameters of adenylate cyclase activity. Since the amounts of adenylate cyclase or BAR per se do not appear to be altered during this process, it was suggested that an 'uncoupling' occurs between BAR and adenylate cyclase during this phase of desensitization. Recovery from this uncoupled state was rapid ($t_{\frac{1}{2}}$ = 7 min) and complete upon removal of the catecholamine from the medium. These results are illustrated in Fig. 1.

The conclusion that an early phase of desensitization involves uncoupling of BAR and adenylate cyclase is also supported by receptor binding studies[11,12]. Work from a number of laboratories suggests that in well coupled BAR/adenylate cyclase systems, agonists bind with high affinity to the receptors in the absence of GTP. In the presence of GTP this high affinity complex does not accumulate and only low affinity binding of agonists is observed. In systems that have been uncoupled by chemical means or by mutational events not only is the capacity of isoproterenol to stimulate adenylate cyclase lost, but agonists bind to BAR with low affinity and there is no effect of guanine nucleotides on agonist binding. The agonist binding properties of BAR of cells that

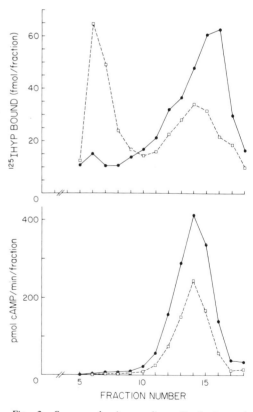

Fig. 2. Sucrose density gradient distribution of β-adrenergic receptors and adenylate cyclase activity after short-term incubation of cells with isoproterenol. Cells were incubated with 1 mM sodium ascorbate (●) or 1 mM sodium ascorbate plus 1 μM isoproterenol (○) for 15 min. The cells were treated with Concanavalin A then lysed and centrifuged in a sucrose density gradient. Upper panel, IHYP was used to determine β-receptor density in gradient fractions. Lower panel, isoproterenol-stimulated adenylate cyclase activity was determined. Taken from Harden et al. 1980.

have been incubated with catecholamines for short periods of time (5–30 min) are similar to those of uncoupled receptors. That is, although there is no change (or only small changes) in the number of receptors, the apparent affinity of isoproterenol for inhibition of IHYP binding is reduced up to ten fold; similarly, there is little effect of GTP on the apparent affinity of isoproterenol[11,12]. The time course of the uncoupling reaction as detected by changes in the affinity of agonist binding is similar to the time course of loss of isoproterenol-stimulated adenylate cyclase activity. Furthermore, the alteration in agonist binding affinity and the reduction of isoproterenol-stimulated adenylate cyclase activity appear to return to control levels with similar time courses upon removal of isoproterenol. The uncoupling reaction exhibits the same concentration–effect relationship for isoproterenol as does stimulation of cAMP accumulation in intact cells. Also, partial agonists (soterenol, zinterol) have roughly equivalent partial effects on the degree of uncoupling and the degree of activation of adenylate cyclase[11].

Although little or no reduction in the density of BAR occurs during a short term incubation of astrocytoma cells with catecholamines, continued exposure to agonist results in a precipitous loss of receptors after 2–4 h[11]. By 24 h the number of BAR and the level of isoproterenol-stimulated enzyme activity are usually reduced to 5–15% of control.

After long-term incubation with catecholamine, recovery of hormone responsiveness or receptor number occurs slowly ($t_{\frac{1}{2}}$ = 14–18 h) upon removal of the catecholamine from the medium (see Fig. 1).

The results of such experiments suggest the following kinetic model for agonist-specific desensitization.

$$BAR_N \rightleftharpoons BAR_U \rightleftharpoons BAR_D$$

The initial process can be envisioned to involve the reversible formation of an altered form of the receptor, BAR_U. Although IHYP still binds to this form of the receptor, the interaction of agonists with BAR_U does not elicit activation of adenylate cyclase.

During a short term incubation with catecholamine, the receptor exists both as BAR_N (native BAR) and BAR_U, and the steady state levels of these two forms are determined by the balance of two reactions. The extent of formation of BAR_U appears to be a function of the concentration of isoproterenol and of the efficacy of partial agonists. With time, the receptor is converted to a form (BAR_D) that is not detected by IHYP; recovery from the BAR_D state is a relatively slow process.

In light of the results described above it is apparent that catecholamine-specific desensitization occurs by a multistep process. Indeed, although the relative rates of the involved reactions may be considerably different, kinetic data would suggest that at least in two astrocytoma cell lines[11], in HC-l hepatoma cells[11], in S-49 lymphoma cells[11,13,14], in frog erythrocytes[12], and in human fibroblasts (unpublished observation), common mechanisms are involved in the development of catecholamine-induced desensitization. That is, catecholamine agonists induce a rapid uncoupling reaction which is followed by another reaction(s) which leads to an apparent loss of BAR from the cell.

Recently it was demonstrated[15] that the uncoupled form of the BAR could be physically separated from the remaining native receptors based on changes in sedimentation properties (Fig. 2). This physical change is rapidly reversible and appears to be associated with the uncoupling reaction. This follows since the uncoupled receptors appear and disappear with the same time course as the onset and reversal of the uncoupling phase of desensitization, the magnitude of the change is the same in both processes (about 50% change in each case), and most importantly, the 'uncoupled' BAR do not exhibit high affinity binding to isoproterenol whereas the remaining native receptors behave as do receptors from naive cells.

An intriguing interpretation of these observations becomes apparent when it is recognized that continued exposure of cells to agonists leads to loss of receptors from the cell. The mechanism underlying the loss of BAR is not known, but an interesting possibility is consistent with a variety of independent observations. First, it is known that down-regulation of plasma membrane receptors for polypeptide hormones involves an agonist-induced endocytotic process[16]. Dansylcadavarin, which blocks the coated pit-mediated endocytosis of polypeptide hormone receptors has been reported also to block the catecholamine-induced loss of BAR in BHK cells[17]. Second, Chuang and Costa[18] reported that 'soluble' BAR could be detected in the cytosol of frog erythrocytes desensitized by exposure to catecholamines. Our observation[15] that up to 60% of the BAR of astrocytoma cells exposed to catecholamines co-migrate in sucrose gradients with enzyme markers for endoplasmic reticulum and golgi apparatus is consistent with the possibility that such uncoupled receptors reside on small endocytotic vesicles. Our most recent studies have shown that the so-called lost BAR (BAR_D) can be completely recovered even in the presence of cycloheximide at a concentration sufficient to block protein synthesis by 90+%. This implies that the modification subserving the $BAR_U \rightarrow BAR_D$ transition does not involve degradation of the BAR polypeptide primary structure. After removal of isoproterenol, recovery of BAR in the presence of cycloheximide begins after a 4 h lag and proceeds to 100% recovery at a rate that is 35–40% that observed in the absence of cycloheximide. Thus, if an endocytotic mechanism is involved in the process of desensitization it apparently does not result in the rapid proteolysis of BAR; perhaps other reversible chemical modifications (glycosylation, phosphorylation?) are involved in the reversible loss of the capacity of BAR to bind to IHYP. It would be premature to conclude from such data that a process of endocytosis and subsequent modification of receptors is involved in agonist-induced down-regulation of BAR. However, a potentially fruitful direction for further study is indicated.

Although some progress has been made in understanding the mechanisms of catecholamine-induced desensitization *in vitro*, the physiological significance of these processes is still not clear. Nonetheless, a growing body of evidence indicates the existence of cellular mechanisms for modification of the number of functional BAR as an adaptive response to fluctuating levels of catecholamines *in vivo*. The study of these processes in model systems may help to provide the details of what appears to be an elaborate set of regulatory processes that modulate catecholamine-mediated intercellular communication.

Reading list

1 Bloom, F. (1975) *Rev. Physiol. Biochem. Pharmacol.* 74, 1–103
2 Perkins, J. P., Su, Y. F. and Harden, T. K. (1979) *Drug Alcohol Dep.* 4, 279–94
3 Daly, J. W. (1977) *Cyclic Nucleotides in the Nervous System*, Plenum Press
4 Kalisker, A., Rutledge, C. O. and Perkins, J. P. (1973) *Mol. Pharmacol.* 9, 619–29
5 Dismukes, R. K. and Daly, J. W. (1975) *Exp. Neurol.* 49, 150–160
6 Wolfe, B. B., Harden, T. K., Sporn, J. R. and Molinoff, P. B. (1978) *J. Pharmacol. Exp. Therap.* 207, 446–57
7 Terasaki, W. L., Brooker, G., deVellis, J., English, D., Hsu, C. Y. and Moylan, R. P. (1978) *Adv. Cyclic Nucleotide Res.* 9, 33–52
8 Lefkowitz, R. J., Wessels, M. R. and Stadel, J. M. (1980) *Curr. Top. Cell. Regul.* Vol. 17, 205–230
9 Mukherjee, C. and Lefkowitz, R. J. (1977) *Mol. Pharmacol.* 13, 291–303
10 Shear, M., Insel, P. A., Melmon, K. L. and Coffino, P. (1976) *J. Biol. Chem.* 251, 7572–7576

11 Su, Y.-F., Harden, T. K. and Perkins, J. P. (1980) *J. Biol. Chem.* 255, 7410–7419
12 Wessels, M. R., Mullikin, D. and Lefkowitz, R. J. (1979) *Mol. Pharmacol.* 16, 10–20
13 Iyengar, R., Bhat, M. K., Riser, M. E. and Birnbaumer, L. (1981) *J. Biol. Chem.* 256, 4810–4815
14 Greene, D. A. and Clark, R. B. (1981) *J. Biol. Chem.* 256, 2105–2108
15 Harden, T. K., Cotton, C. U., Waldon, G. L., Lutton, J. K. and Perkins, J. P. (1980) *Science*, 210, 441–443
16 Pastan, I. H. and Willingham, M. C. (1981) *Ann. Rev. Physiol.* 43, 239–250
17 Reggiani, A., Vernaleone, F. and Robison, G. A. (1980) *Neurosci. Abstr.* 6, 534
18 Chuang, D. M. and Costa, E. (1979) *Proc. Natl Acad. Aci. U.S.A.* 76, 3024–3028

Proving a role for cyclic AMP in synaptic transmission

Clark A. Briggs and Donald A. McAfee

Division of Neurosciences, City of Hope Research Institute, Duarte, CA 91010, U.S.A.

While the relationships are obvious, few scientists appreciate the large degree to which endocrine and nervous systems overlap in their mechanisms and functions. After all, neurons and endocrine cells each release a signal molecule that diffuses to the target cell and there binds with a specific receptor. Indeed, adrenaline and noradrenaline are signal molecules employed by both systems. Endocrine cells are clustered into a few glands that secrete into the circulation which, in turn, conveys the molecule to all tissues including the target tissue. The neuron, on the other hand, extends a cellular process containing the secretory mechanism and signal molecule to the target cell. Thus, the differences between these two systems may be more a matter of form than substance.

Commonly, the distinction is one of metabolic v. electrical events, of slow v. fast control. Certainly, the electrical events of excitable membranes are impressive and can, in the short term, occur independently of cellular metabolism. Nevertheless, most neurobiologists would concede that even these events are eventually modulated by metabolic processes, and that long-term changes, such as those involving learning and memory, are totally dependent upon metabolism.

It was an endocrinologist, Earl Sutherland, and his colleagues, who provided neurobiologists with a potentially powerful link between a signal molecule, a membrane event and metabolism[1]. A dozen years ago an issue of importance among endocrinologists was how impermeable hormones such as adrenaline and peptides could influence cellular metabolism. Neurobiologists, on the other hand, readily accepted the idea that the neurotransmitters acted externally on membrane-bound receptors to control immediate membrane events, but lacked adequate models for long-term changes in excitability. None should be astonished, then, at the fervor with which Sutherland's second messenger concept was accepted and applied in both endocrinology and neurobiology (Fig. 1). Regardless of how the signal molecule is delivered to the receptor there is initiated a sequence of enzyme reactions beginning with adenylate cyclase and culminating in the hormone or post-synaptic effect (Fig. 2).

The literature on cyclic nucleotides in the nervous system is immense and is regularly reviewed in a comprehensive manner[2-11]. Our purpose here is to present only a brief and opinionated commentary from the experimentalist's point of view. We will consider only the hypothesis: cyclic AMP mediates the effect of neurotransmitters at certain neuron–neuron synapses.

Criteria for a cyclic AMP hypothesis

Using the model in Fig. 1, one could set out a list of criteria to test the hypothesis that the effects of a neurotransmitter are mediated by cyclic AMP[2]. (1) Clearly, the neurotransmitter should specifically activate a receptor-coupled *adenylate cyclase* in neuron membrane preparations. (2) It would follow that *synaptic activity* should augment cyclic AMP levels and then increase *protein phosphorylation* prior to the physiological response. (3) One should be able to bypass the neurotransmitter altogether and *mimic* the physiological response with intracellular injections of cyclic AMP or the protein kinase. (4) *Pharmacological agents* which alter accumulation of cyclic AMP should similarly alter the synaptic response. Agents which modify neurotransmitter receptor activation should similarly alter cyclic AMP synthesis and protein phosphorylation. (5) Since nervous tissue is heterogeneous it is important to show that the *biochemical* responses are *localized* to the cells showing cyclic AMP-dependent *physiological* responses.

Each criterion can be approached experimentally but the exercise is not at all trivial, especially in the nervous system. A receptor-coupled cyclase is essential to the second messenger hypothesis, but cyclic nucleotides may be regulated by intracellular Ca^{2+} and GTP. Adenylate cyclases coupled to adenosine (A_2), β-adrenergic, dopamine (D_1), and serotonin receptors are the best characterized of many identified in membrane preparations from nervous tissue[2,12]. The heterogeneity of membrane preparations from nervous tissue precludes the distinction of synaptic from extrasynaptic or even extraneuronal cyclase. Rigorous quantitative pharmacology is required in equating the receptor coupled to the cyclase with the receptor utilized in synaptic transmission. Unfortunately, the application of this pharmacology, when available, is too often superficial.

The advent of reliable radioimmunoassay kits has greatly simplified the measurement of cyclic nucleotides. But, it has never been made clear how much of an increase in cyclic AMP is necessary in order to induce the synaptic response, even though large changes are considered more interesting than small changes. An increase in cyclic AMP content following exposure of the tissue to a putative neurotransmitter is too frequently hailed as evidence that

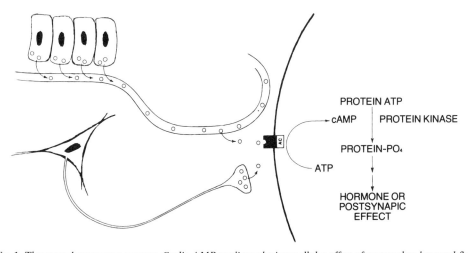

Fig. 1. The second messenger concept. Cyclic AMP mediates the intracellular effect of neuronal or humoral first messengers. Here, cyclic AMP acts as a cofactor for a protein kinase. In hepatic glycogenolysis, phosphorylation activates phosphorylase kinase and inactivates glycogen synthetase. Little is known of the action of phosphorylated proteins at the synapse, but speculation abounds (see Fig. 2).

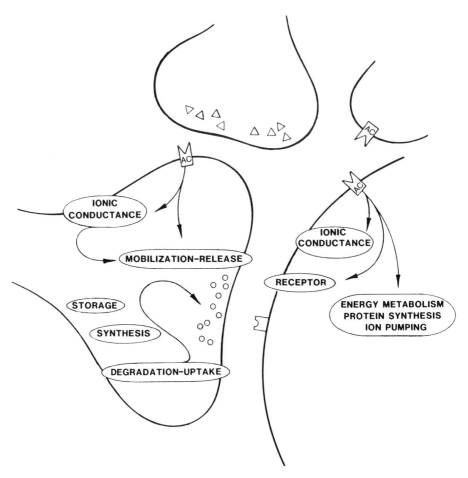

Fig. 2. A functional schematic of the synaptic region. Adenylate cyclase coupled to presynaptic receptors may control the release of neurotransmitters by regulating any number of possible neurotransmitter release processes. Similarly, post-synaptic membrane excitability or cellular metabolism could be controlled by neurotransmitter or neurohumoral first messengers. Perisynaptic glial elements may regulate synaptic efficacy by uptake and metabolism of neurotransmitters. In nervous tissue, cyclic AMP may mediate the effects of neurotransmitters and hormones not only in neurons but also in glia and the smooth muscle of blood vessels.

cyclic AMP mediates the synaptic response. Exogenous neurotransmitter agonists could raise cyclic AMP at non-synaptic and even non-neuronal sites[6]. Immunohistochemistry can be used to localize and even semi-quantitate cyclic nucleotides in specific cell types. However, the detected cyclic nucleotide may belong only to that subset which somehow remains bound or trapped during the extensive incubation and washing of the frozen tissue sections. Clearly, the most important kind of observation is that *synaptic* activity raises cyclic AMP levels in the tissue, but this observation has been made only in the cerebellum[7,11], sympathetic ganglion[6], and in *Aplysia* abdominal ganglion[4] and bag cell clusters[3].

It is believed that probably all effects of cyclic nucleotides are brought about by protein phosphorylation; only the protein kinases are known to be physiologically regulated simply by the binding of a cyclic nucleotide. Characterization of synaptic phosphorylation is a very difficult task, but Greengard's laboratory has succeeded in identifying a neuron-specific protein (Protein I) which is a substrate for both a cyclic AMP-dependent kinase and a calmodulin-dependent kinase[2]. These exciting observations provide a clear molecular basis for the synergism often suspected between Ca^{2+} and cyclic nucleotides. Protein I (actually two similar proteins, Ia and Ib) is found in many synapses and in association with synaptic vesicles, but its role in synaptic activity is unknown. Exogenous serotonin and dopamine can increase cyclic AMP-dependent phosphorylation of Protein I in the facial motor nucleus and in the superior cervical ganglion[2]. Recently, it has been demonstrated that preganglionic stimulation increases the phosphorylation of Protein I[13]. It will be interesting to know whether synaptically-released neurotransmitter can control the cyclic AMP-dependent phosphorylation of Protein I.

The criterion of mimicry is not a powerful test of the cyclic AMP hypothesis unless the underlying mechanisms of the transmitter response are known in some detail. All drugs could be classified into three categories: those that *inhibit*, those that *excite*, and those that *do nothing*. By chance alone, cyclic AMP could appear to mimic a neurotransmitter in a third of the preparations where the synaptic action is described in the simple terms of excitability. Cyclic AMP acts physiologically at intracellular sites, but it is more convenient to apply cyclic AMP analogs extracellularly. Controls must be made for effects on adenosine receptors, pH, and release of endogenous neuroactive substances. The 8-substituted derivatives of cyclic AMP are useful analogs because they are more lipophilic, less sensitive to phosphodiesterase, and not metabolized to an adenosine receptor agonist[11].

A major problem in this field is the lack of good pharmacological studies and tools. Too few investigators do dose–response or specificity studies. Phosphodiesterase inhibitors, such as papaverine and the methylxanthines, have significant effects on Ca^{2+} metabolism and are potent antagonists at the adenosine receptor[10,12]; Ro20-1724 appears to be a more specific phosphodiesterase inhibitor. There is no specific antagonist of adenylate cyclase independent of the receptor blockers, but GTP and forskolin may specifically activate this enzyme in a reversible fashion[12,14]. There are no specific, membrane-permeable agents directed towards the kinases or phosphatases. One can only wistfully wish for greater pharmacological control over the system.

Model systems

Vertebrate central nervous systems

The clearest picture of a role for cyclic AMP in vertebrate synaptic transmission has been presented for the cerebellum[7,11]. Histological studies indicate that the Purkinje neuron of the cerebellum receives a noradrenergic innervation from the locus coeruleus. Stimulation of this synapse or application of noradrenaline decreases the rate of action potential discharge and increases the immunohistochemical staining for cyclic AMP in Purkinje neurons. A β-adrenergic receptor is responsible for the electrophysiological effect. The cerebellum, like other nervous and non-nervous tissues, contains an adenylate cyclase coupled to a β-adrenergic receptor; it is assumed that this receptor is responsible for regulating cyclic AMP in the Purkinje neuron. Phosphodiesterase inhibitors potentiate both the effect of synaptic stimulation and exogenous noradrenaline on Purkinje neuron discharge. These inhibitors can themselves depress the discharge. Cyclic AMP appears to mimic the effects of noradrenaline and locus coeruleus stimulation, but little is known about the ionic mechanisms responsible for the inhibition of discharge by these procedures.

Superior cervical sympathetic ganglia

The sympathetic ganglion with its well-defined input (preganglionic) and output (post-ganglionic) nerves is a good choice as a model system for the metabolic dependence of synaptic transmission. The synaptic organization consists primarily of a powerful nicotinic cholinergic (depolarizing) synapse at the preganglionic termination on the post-ganglionic neuron. However, there are several lines of evidence that suggest that post-ganglionic neurons also receive a dopaminergic synapse from a small intensely fluorescent interneuron (SIF cell). According to the SIF cell hypothesis, this dopaminergic synapse generates a slow inhibitory post-synaptic potential (slow-IPSP) and the SIF cell, in turn, receives an excitatory muscarinic synaptic input from preganglionic terminals. Our hypothesis, based upon the SIF cell hypothesis, was that the action of dopamine and hence the slow-IPSP was mediated by cyclic AMP. This attractive model was subjected to testing by the criteria listed above[6].

Dopamine-sensitive adenylate cyclase activity was first demonstrated in the bovine ganglion, though it has not been subsequently demonstrated in rat or rabbit ganglia. However, preganglionic stimulation of the rat and rabbit ganglia (60 s at 10 Hz) caused a two-fold increase in cyclic AMP, and this increase was antagonized by the same agents which were reported to block the slow-IPSP. Similarly, muscarinic agonists raised cyclic AMP levels two-fold. This appeared to be due to activation of a dopaminergic interneuron because the muscarinic effect was inhibited by low Ca^{2+} and α-adrenergic antagonists.

We were surprised that exogenous dopamine raised cyclic AMP only slightly (15%) and we have encountered other problems with interpretation of electrophysiological correlates and specificity of pharmacological agents. Initial experiments using extracellular recording techniques (sucrose gap) demonstrated well-defined slow synaptic potentials and dopamine hyperpolarizations potentiated by theophylline, a phosphodiesterase inhibitor. Cyclic AMP hyperpolarized post-ganglionic neurons, but only weakly. In later years, the more powerful intracellular techniques did not demonstrate well-defined slow synaptic potentials. However, these techniques did show theophylline to non-specifically activate Ca^{2+}-dependent potentials, dopamine to hyperpolarize by weakly activating α-receptors, and cyclic AMP to be degraded to a hyperpolarizing adenosine receptor agonist. Our evidence is that at least the electrogenic actions of α- and adenosine-receptors are not mediated by cyclic AMP[6]. However, Ashe and Libet have recently presented evidence that cyclic AMP could mediate an hours long potentiation of slow synaptic potentials following activation of a dopamine (D_1) receptor[15]. Thus, the sympathetic ganglion continues as a model system for testing cyclic nucleotide hypotheses.

Invertebrate neurons

Many neuronal somata in the CNS of *Aplysia* are large, and specific neurons can be visually identified from preparation to preparation. Biochemical as well as electrophysiological techniques can be applied to single neurons. Levitan[16], Treistman[17] and co-workers have indicated that cyclic AMP mediates an increase in K^+ conductance which appears to be involved in long-term inhibition of the neuron R15. While the transmitter secreted into this inhibitory synapse is not known, the inhibitory effect of branchial nerve stimulation is mimicked by cyclic AMP, a GTP analog, and serotonin. In other model neurons cyclic AMP appears to mediate a decrease in K^+ conductance[3,4,18].

Cyclic AMP is the subject of intense study in two laboratories, Strumwasser's and Kandel's, which have for some time combined neurochemical and neurophysiological approaches to the study of behavior. Egg-laying behavior in *Aplysia* is dependent upon a long-lasting (30 min) burst of activity in the neuroendocrine bag cells. This long discharge is induced by only a brief synaptic input. Cyclic AMP levels and protein phosphorylation in bag cells increase during the first minute of discharge and cyclic AMP analogs mimic the synaptic input[3]. Injection of cyclic AMP-dependent protein kinase (catalytic subunit) into bag cells reproduced some of the effects of exogenous cyclic AMP and synaptic activity, apparently by reducing the K^+ conductance[3].

The most complete story concerning a role for cyclic AMP in synaptic transmission has been presented by Kandel and colleagues[4]. It is possible to demonstrate a long-term facilitation of the gill withdrawal reflex in a learning paradigm. This behavior is associated with presynaptic facilitation of the sensory neuron synapse with the motor neuron. The ionic basis of this facilitation is the potentiation of a Ca^{2+} current, and thus the Ca^{2+} influx associated with the action potential, by the inhibition of a K^+ conductance[19]. The facilitory transmitter is unknown, but serotonin (and not other biogenic amines) mimics the synaptically-induced facilitation. Serotonin, dopamine, and synaptic activity increase cyclic AMP levels in abdominal ganglia and in isolated neuronal somata. Phosphodiesterase inhibitors applied extracellularly and cyclic AMP injected into the sensory neuron increase the voltage-dependent Ca^{2+} current, decrease membrane conductance, and facilitate release. Cyclic AMP-dependent protein kinase (catalytic subunit) injected into the sensory neuron mimics the effects of injected cyclic AMP[20]. While protein kinase is relatively non-specific the above two approaches are important in constructing the molecular framework underlying biochemical control of neuronal excitability.

Concluding remarks

This has been a brief overview of the question: does cyclic AMP mediate a synaptic response? One may be surprised that, after a dozen years and a vast literature, our knowledge is no more than half-vast. During this time we have learned much about cyclic AMP metabolism. However, progress has been limited because too little is known about the ionic mechanisms underlying synaptic responses. As we learn more about receptors, we find that our pharmacological tools are inadequate. Lastly, little is known about the relationships between protein phosphorylation and neuronal excitability, yet this is a fundamental tenet of the cyclic nucleotide hypothesis. We think it is in this area where some of the most exciting progress will occur in the next decade.

Acknowledgements

We gratefully thank Lloyd E. Carder II for preparing the figures, and Drs B. Henon, M. Kennedy, J. Ono, G. Stone and F. Strumwasser for their many helpful comments.

Reading list

1 Robison, G. A., Butcher, R. W. and Sutherland, E. W. (1971) *Cyclic AMP*, Academic Press, New York
2 Greengard, P. *The Harvey Lecture Series*, Academic Press, New York (in press)
3 Strumwasser, F., Kaczmarek, L. K., Jennings, K. R. and Chiu, A. Y. (1981) in *Neurosecretion, Molecules, Cells and Systems* (Lederis, K. and Farner, D. S., eds), pp. 251–270, Plenum Press, New York
4 Klein, M., Shapiro, E. and Kandel, E. R. (1980) *J. Exp. Biol.* 89, 117–157
5 Kupfermann, I. (1980) *Annu. Rev. Physiol.* 42, 629–641
6 McAfee, D. A., Henon, B. K., Whiting, G. J., Horn, J. P., Yarowsky, P. J. and Turner, D. K. (1980) *Fed. Proc. Fed. Am. Soc. Exp. Biol.* 39, 2997–3002
7 Standaert, F. G. (1979) *Fed. Proc. Fed. Am. Soc. Exp. Biol. (Symp.)* 38, 2182–2217
8 Nathanson, J. A. (1977) *Physiol. Rev.* 57, 157–256

9 Phyllis, J. W. (1977) *Can. J. Neurol. Sci.* 4, 153–195
10 Tsien, R. W. (1977) *Adv. Cyclic Nucleotide Res.* 8, 363–420
11 Bloom, F. E. (1975) *Rev. Physiol. Biochem. Pharmacol.* 74, 1–103
12 Daly, J. W., Bruns, R. F. and Snyder, S. H. (1981) *Life Sci.* 28, 2083–2097
13 Nestler, E. R. and Greengard, P. (1981) *Soc. Neurosci. Abstr.* 7, 707
14 Seamon, K. B., Padgett, W. and Daly, J. W. (1981) *Proc. Natl Acad. Sci. U.S.A.* 78, 3363–3367
15 Ashe, J. H. and Libet, B. (1981) *Brain Res.* 217, 93–106
16 Adams, W. B., Parnas, I. and Levitan, I. B. (1980) *J. Neurophysiol.* 44, 1148–1160
17 Treistman, S. N. (1981) *Science*, 211, 59–61
18 Deterre, P., Paupardin-Tritsch, D., Bockaert, J. and Gerschenfeld, H. M. (1981) *Nature (London)*, 290, 783–785
19 Klein, M. and Kandel, E. R. (1980) *Proc. Natl Acad. Sci. U.S.A.* 77, 6912–6916
20 Castellucci, V. F., Kandel, E. R., Schwartz, J. H., Wilson, F. D., Nairn, A. C. and Greengard, P. (1980) *Proc. Natl Acad. Sci. U.S.A.* 77, 7492–7496

Cyclic nucleotides and the nervous system

Tamas Bartfai

Department of Biochemistry, Arrhenius Laboratory, University of Stockholm, S-106 91 Stockholm, Sweden.

Major classes of drugs such as antipsychotics, antidepressants and antihypertensives profoundly influence the cyclic nucleotide systems.

Cyclic nucleotides have been implicated as second messengers for hormones and neurotransmitters in the regulation of metabolic activities, cell division and cell differentiation[1,2]. The role of cAMP and cGMP as second messengers in the nervous system has been extensively studied in the last decade[1,2]. The main impetus for these studies came from the demonstration of the inhibitory action of the antipsychotic drugs on the dopamine-activated adenylate cyclase in the striatum[3]. Studies on the sympathetic ganglion implicated cAMP and cGMP as second messengers in dopaminergic and muscarinic cholinergic action, respectively[4]. The pharmacological importance of cyclic nucleotides becomes obvious if one considers that most antipsychotic, antidepressant and antihypertensive drugs affect dopaminergic, serotonergic and noradrenergic neurotransmission, which at D_1-dopamine receptors, serotonin-receptors and β-receptors respectively involves cAMP as second messenger (cf. Fig. 1 for drugs effecting cyclic nucleotide levels). In the present review some recent examples of the synaptic effects of those neurotransmitters and drugs which involve cyclic nucleotides are given.

The mechanism of action of cyclic nucleotides: a cascade

Studies in nervous and non-nervous tissues indicate that cyclic nucleotide dependent reactions involve several steps as outlined below.

Step 1. cAMP is generated by a unique membrane bound enzyme, adenylate cyclase, which can be activated by a number

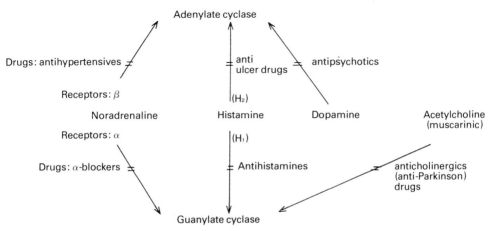

Fig. 1. Activation of adenylate and guanylate cyclases by some neurotransmitters and some representative classes of drugs which act as antagonists and thereby affect cAMP or cGMP production.

of neurotransmitters and hormones[1-3] (Fig. 1).

Step 2. cAMP combines with high affinity (K_d = 0.01–0.05 μM) with the cAMP-dependent protein kinase, which dissociates into a cAMP-regulatory subunit complex and active catalytic subunits.

Step 3. The active catalytic subunit of protein kinase phosphorylates specific proteins. The phosphorylation state of certain membrane proteins may then regulate the permeability of the membrane.

Step 4. The phosphorylated membrane proteins are rapidly dephosphorylated by protein phosphatases.

Step 5. The cellular levels of cAMP are also rapidly reduced to the basal level via hydrolysis by the cAMP-phosphodiesterase (PDE).

cGMP is generated by the guanylate cyclase which occurs in membrane bound and soluble form and which can be activated in whole cells by a number of neurotransmitters (Fig. 1)[5]. The elevated cGMP levels lead to activation of the cGMP-dependent protein kinases and subsequent phosphorylation of specific proteins. These in turn can be dephosphorylated by protein phosphatases. The elevated cGMP levels are reduced by the action of the cGMP-PDE[5].

It should be noted that although the mechanism of action of the two cyclic nucleotide activated systems is similar, the cAMP- and cGMP-dependent reactions involve specific receptors coupled to adenylate cyclase or guanylate cyclase, respectively; e.g. H_2-histamine receptor-stimulation of cAMP and H_1-histamine receptor-stimulation of cGMP synthesis, respectively. The cAMP- and cGMP-dependent protein kinases are distinct proteins with specific protein substrates which are dephosphorylated by endogenous protein phosphatases. Degradation of cAMP and cGMP is also carried out via specific enzymes. All of the enzymes involved in cyclic nucleotide metabolism have been shown to occur with high specific activity in nervous tissues. Several phosphoprotein targets of cAMP- and cGMP-dependent protein kinases[1,2] which are specific for nervous tissues have been discovered and it is likely that these are intimately involved in those synaptic actions where cyclic nucleotides play a role[1,2].

In most regions of the nervous system basal levels of cAMP are ten-fold higher than those of cGMP, and only under very special conditions will activation occur of cAMP-dependent protein kinase by cGMP or degradation of cAMP by the cGMP-phosphodiesterase. It is therefore possible to design drugs which affect only events involving cAMP or cGMP.

Drug action on the cascade

Drugs may interfere at any one of the five major steps indicated above, and thereby influence the phosphorylation level of a specific phosphoprotein which is involved in the physiological action of a neurotransmitter.

Step 1. Most commonly, drugs that affect the cAMP-dependent protein phosphorylation system do so by a direct action on the receptors preventing the activation of adenylate cyclase by the neurotransmitter (cf. Fig. 1). The inhibitory action of antipsychotic drugs on the dopamine-mediated activation of adenylate cyclase or of the β-blocker propranolol on the noradrenaline-mediated activation of the adenylate cyclase may serve as representative examples. It is important to note in this context not only that blockade of activation of adenylate cyclase may occur but also that persistent activation of the enzyme may take place. Such activation appears to be the mode of action of cholera toxin[6].

Steps 2–4. There are no specific drugs which interfere with the cAMP-mediated activation of the protein kinase: however, an endogenous, heat-stable inhibitor of the protein kinase is known[7]. Furthermore, an important action of steroid hormones may be their effect on protein phosphoryl-

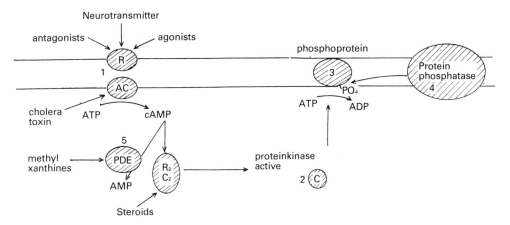

Fig. 2. Site of action of some drugs which affect cyclic nucleotide protein phosphorylation systems at the cell membrane and inside the cell. The numbers refer to the reaction steps of the cascade as described in the text.

ation, which is exerted through regulation of the activity (autophosphorylation) of the cAMP-dependent protein kinase[1,2]. There are no specific drugs known for promotion or inhibition of the protein dephosphorylation.

Step 5. There are several drugs known which inhibit the 3'5' cyclic nucleotide phosphodiesterase and thereby prolong elevated cyclic nucleotide levels and increase the probability of the phosphorylation of the various phosphoproteins. The most common inhibitors of PDE are the methylxanthines, such as theophylline and caffeine. Several of the numerous pharmacological actions of these drugs may be ascribed to inhibition of PDE while others involve interactions with adenosine receptors. It should be mentioned that in the retina a light activated cGMP-PDE occurs. Thus here, the cyclic nucleotide level (and protein phosphorylation state) is influenced through regulation of a degrading enzyme (PDE) while in most other systems it is the synthesis of the cyclic nucleotide which is controlled by external stimuli (neurotransmitters).

The mechanism of action of hormones and neurotransmitters which involves cyclic nucleotides was elucidated in peripheral non-nervous and nervous tissues and the above discussed cascades are much alike in nervous and non-nervous tissues. The second part of this review gives some recent examples of involvement of cyclic nucleotides in specific neuronal interactions which take place at both sides of the synapse.

Presynaptic actions involving cyclic nucleotides

Neurotransmitter synthesis

As demonstrated earlier, increased impulse flow in noradrenergic neurons leads to activation of tyrosine hydroxylase via a cAMP-dependent phosphorylation[1,2]. In this way presynaptic β-receptors which stimulate cAMP synthesis appear to stimulate the synthesis of catecholamine neurotransmitters.

Neurotransmitter release facilitation

In the abdominal ganglion of *Aplysia*, serotonin facilitates release of neurotransmitter from a sensory neuron onto a follower neuron. Injection of cAMP into the presynaptic nerve terminal of the sensory neuron, which carries the serotonin receptors, showed that cAMP mimics facilitation of neurotransmitter release by serotonin. Furthermore it could be shown that this action of cAMP is mediated via activation of a cAMP-dependent protein kinase since injection of the active protein kinase catalytic subunit caused facilitation of neurotransmitter release from the sensory neuron and thus mimicked the action of serotonin[8].

In the sympathetic neurons of guinea pig vas deferens, where microinjection of cAMP or the active protein kinase into the nerve terminal is not yet feasible, one can demonstrate that a permeant analogue of cAMP, 8-Br-cAMP, enhances the electrical stimulation-evoked release of noradrenaline[9]. This action mimics the effect of β-receptor agonists (e.g. noradrenaline).

Inhibition

Muscarinic agonists acting at autoreceptors inhibit release of acetylcholine from hippocampal cholinergic nerve endings in the rat. This effect of muscarinic agonists could be mimicked by permeant cGMP analogues, 8-Br-cGMP and dibutyryl-cGMP, or by incubation with nitrosoamines which activate the guanylate cyclase[10].

It appears from electrophysiological experiments in *Aplysia* and from $^{45}Ca^{2+}$-uptake experiments with synaptosomes from rat brain that facilitation and inhibition of neurotransmitter release by cAMP and cGMP respectively may involve promotion and inhibition of Ca^{2+} influx into the nerve terminal, respectively.

Post-synaptic actions involving cyclic nucleotides

There are extensive reviews on the post-synaptic actions mediated by cyclic nucleotides as second messenger[1,2]. Some examples are presented here.

Purkinje cell firing is inhibited by activation of non-adrenergic neurons which form synapses with the noradrenergic cells. It was shown by iontophoretic techniques that the action of noradrenaline at β-receptors can be mimicked by iontophoresis of cAMP onto the Purkinje cells[1,2].

Several studies have shown good correlation between the relaxation of smooth muscle mediated by nitroglycerin and other nitrocompounds (which activate cGMP synthesis) and relaxation caused by cGMP analogues.

Trans-synaptic effects

There is increasing evidence to indicate that reduction of cyclic nucleotide levels involves not only the action of PDE but also the extrusion of the cyclic nucleotide from the cell[11]. One example is the avian erythrocyte which lacks PDE and pumps out cAMP which is formed upon β-receptor stimulation. Neuroblastoma cells can release cGMP; also, release of cGMP from the pineal gland has been reported. If, as appears to be the case, protein kinases on the cell surface of other cells exist, these may use the extracellular cyclic nucleotide as a signal. The possibility that extensive stimulation in some pathological instances may lead to overflow of cyclic nucleotides is not at all remote since, for example, cholera toxin persistently activates adenylate cyclase[6]. Repetitive discharge in an epileptic focus may raise cGMP levels 10–50 fold above normal levels as indicated by large increases in cGMP levels upon repetitive depolarizations in the presence of extracellular Ca^{2+}. In both of these instances the activity of PDE may not suffice to reduce cAMP and cGMP levels respectively in which case overflow of the cyclic nucleotide may well occur.

Conclusions

Although very few drugs are designed to affect the cyclic nucleotide/protein phosphorylation system in nervous tissue, several major classes of drugs do act through an indirect effect on this system.

Some drugs act primarily at the cell surface, like many effective antipsychotic drugs which are dopamine antagonists, and the antidepressants which affect uptake and thereby stimulation of receptors for monoamines. It should be kept in mind, however, that supersensitivity and subsensitivity to these drugs may not be confined to the increase or decrease in the number of the respective receptors but may also involve changes in the activity of all enzymes (adenylate cyclase, protein kinase, protein phosphatase and PDE) of the cascade.

Several other agents, including steroids and methylxanthines, affect the cascade at intracellular sites such as the activity of the protein kinase and the activity of PDE.

New drugs may affect physiological responses by directly reacting with the specific phosphoproteins involved.

Reading list

1 Greengard, P. (1978) *Cyclic Nucleotides, Phosphorylated Proteins and Neuronal Function*, Raven Press, New York
2 Kebabian, J. W. (1977) *Adv. Cyclic. Nucleotide Res.* 8, 421–508
3 Clement-Cormier, Y. C., Kebabian, J. W., Petzold, G. L. and Greengard, P. (1974) *Proc. Natl Acad. Sci. U.S.A.* 71, 1113–1117
4 McAfee, D. A. and Greengard, P. (1972) *Science*, 178, 310–312
5 Goldberg, N. D. and Haddox, M. K. (1978) *Annu. Rev. Biochem.* 46, 823–896
6 Johnson, G. L., Kaslow, M. R. and Bourne, H. R. (1978) *Proc. Natl Acad. Sci. U.S.A.* 75, 3113–3117
7 Walsh, D. A., Ashby, C. D., Gonzalez, C., Calkins, D., Fischer, E. H. and Krebs, E. G. (1971) *J. Biol. Chem.* 246, 1977–1985
8 Castelucci, V. F., Kandel, E. R., Schwartz, J. C., Wilson, F. D., Nairn, A. C. and Greengard, P. (1980) *Proc. Natl Acad. Sci. U.S.A.* 77, 7492–7496
9 Stjärne, L., Bartfai, T. and Alberts, P. (1979) *Naunyn-Schmiedebergs Arch. Pharmakol.* 308, 99–105
10 Nordström, Ö. and Bartfai, T. (1981) *Brain Res.* 213, 467–471
11 Bartfai, T. (1980) in *Current Topics of Cellular Regulation* (Horecher, B. L. and Stadtman, E. R., eds), Vol. 16, pp. 226–269

Molecular mechanisms involved in α-adrenergic responses

John H. Exton

Laboratories for the Studies of Metabolic Disorders, Howard Hughes Medical Institute and Department of Physiology, Vanderbilt University School of Medicine, Nashville, TN 37232 U.S.A.

There are two basic types of α-adrenergic receptor (α_1 and α_2) which differ in their selectivity for the antagonists prazosin and yohimbine, and the agonists clonidine and α-methylnorepinephrine. α_1-Receptors are located post-synaptically and their activation leads to changes in cell Ca^{2+} fluxes which apparently result in a rise in cytosolic Ca^{2+}. The changes may involve influx of extracellular Ca^{2+} through Ca^{2+} 'gates' in the plasma membrane, or release of Ca^{2+} from intracellular organelles such as mitochondria. There is an accompanying increase in the turnover of phosphatidylinositol, which may play a role in the Ca^{2+} changes. The rise in cytosolic Ca^{2+} is believed to be responsible for the physiological responses, and it has been hypothesized that the phosphorylation of specific enzymes and proteins by a Ca^{2+}-calmodulin-dependent protein kinase(s) may be involved. α_2-Receptors may be located presynaptically where they mediate feedback inhibition of norepinephrine release, or post-synaptically where their activation results in a decrease in cAMP to which many of the physiological changes can be attributed. The reduction in cAMP is due to inhibition of adenylate cyclase. It has been hypothesized that GTP and an inhibitory guanine nucleotide-binding protein are involved in coupling the α_2-receptor to the catalytic moiety of adenylate cyclase.

Classification of α-adrenergic receptors

The characteristics of α-adrenergic receptors have recently been described in this journal by Lefkowitz and Hoffman[1], and will therefore be reviewed only briefly in this article. It is clear that there are two basic types of α-receptor designated α_1 and α_2. α_1-Receptors are located post-synaptically, are blocked more potently by prazosin than by yohimbine, and generally have low affinity for the agonists clonidine and α-methylnorepinephrine. On the other hand, α_2-receptors are located both pre- and post-synaptically, are blocked potently by yohimbine and have high affinity for clonidine and α-methylnorepinephrine. An additional distinguishing feature proposed by Lefkowitz[1] is that guanine nucleotides decrease the agonist affinity of α_2-receptors, but not of α_1-receptors. However, it is not certain how general this distinction is.

There are many compounds which are relatively non-selective for the two types of receptor including epinephrine, norepinephrine and ergot alkaloids. In addition, some heterogeneity exists within each subclass and the above characteristics may vary from tissue to tissue. Furthermore, many tissues or cells contain both types of α-receptors.

Mechanisms involved in α_2-adrenergic responses in platelets

Presynaptic α_2-receptors mediate feedback inhibition of norepinephrine release from noradrenergic nerve endings, whereas post-synaptic α_2 receptors are involved in other responses such as platelet aggregation and inhibition of insulin secretion. Post-synaptic α_2-receptors appear to have in common the property of lowering intracellular cAMP through inhibition of adenylate cyclase (Table I)[2]. This has been demonstrated most clearly in human and rabbit platelets, and accounts for the stimulation of platelet aggregation by α-agonists. In these cells, epinephrine, norepinephrine and α-methylnorepinephrine inhibit adenylate cyclase under basal conditions or when the enzyme is stimulated by agonists such as prostaglandin E_1. This inhibition is increased by β-blockers and is potently inhibited by ergot alkaloids, yohimbine, and imidazoline derivatives such as clonidine and phentolamine. The receptor mediating inhibition of the cyclase thus exhibits most of the properties expected for the α_2-type. This conclusion is supported by studies of the binding of [^{3}H]dihydroergocryptine, [^{3}H]dihydroergonine and [^{3}H]phentolamine to platelet membranes which yield results generally similar to those found for adenylate cyclase inhibition.

Based on the finding that yohimbine, phentolamine, norepinephrine, methoxamine and prazosin monotonically inhibit [^{3}H]dihydroergocryptine binding to human platelets, it has been concluded that the α-receptors of these cells are exclusively of the α_2-type[1]. Analogous to findings with β-receptors, guanine nucleotides have been observed to decrease the affinity of platelet α_2-receptors for agonists, but not antagonists[1,3]. Michel et al.[3] have proposed that the α_2-receptors exist in two affinity states and that guanine nucleotides convert the high affinity receptors to a low affinity state. High concentrations of Na^+ also reduce the affinity of the receptors, but the effect is exerted on both receptor states[3].

Jakobs and co-workers[2] have shown that α-adrenergic inhibition of platelet adenylate cyclase requires GTP. The inhibition is not only observed under basal conditions, but also when the enzyme is activated by prostaglandin E_1, β-agonists, fluoride and cholera toxin[2]. However, when the enzyme is fully activated by 'stable' GTP analogues such as GMP-P(NH)P, GMP-P(CH$_2$)P and GTP-γ-S, it is not susceptible to inhibition by epinephrine in the absence or presence of GTP[2]. Likewise, GMP-P(NH)P, GMP-P(CH$_2$)P and GTP-γ-S can reverse the inhibitory action of epinephrine plus GTP on the enzyme. Based on these observations, Jakobs et al.[2] have proposed that α-adrenergic inhibition of platelet adenylate cyclase results from enhanced inactiva-

TABLE I. Tissues in which α_2-receptors have been identified and linked to inhibition of cAMP formation

Tissue	α_2-Receptors identified by radioligand binding	α-Agonist-mediated inhibition of adenylate cyclase or cAMP accumulation shown
Platelets	+	+*
Adipose	+	+*
Liver	+	+*
Salivary	+	+
Heart	+	+
Pancreatic Islets	−	+
Thyroid	−	+
Glia	−	+
Brain	+	−
Parathyroid	−	+
Kidney	+	−
Uterus	+	−
Bladder (amphibian)	−	+
Skin (amphibian)	−	+

*Shown to be α_2 response

tion of the catalytically active form of the enzyme and have suggested that this might involve stimulation of the GTPase linked to the adenylate cyclase system.

Jakobs et al.[2] and Steer and Wood[4] have presented evidence that the GTP-dependent component involved in the α-inhibition of platelet adenylate cyclase is different from that mediating the stimulatory effect of prostaglandin E_1. The principal evidence is that inhibition is only seen with GTP at micromolar concentrations, whereas stimulation is observed with much lower concentrations. The existence of two distinct guanine nucleotide regulatory components in platelets would be compatible with observations in other tissues.

α_2-Adrenergic responses in other tissues

α-Adrenergic inhibition of adenylate cyclase has been reported for other tissues including adipose tissue, liver, neuroblastoma-glioma hybrid cells and parotid gland (Table I)[2]. In general, the inhibition in these tissues is similar to that of the platelet system, i.e. it is mediated by α_2-receptors and requires GTP. One apparent difference from human platelets is that monovalent cations are needed for the effect: these ions activate the enzyme in the presence of GTP and the activation is inhibited by α_2-agonists.

α-Agonists have also been reported to lower cAMP levels in pancreatic islets, bladder, frog skin, thyroid, glial cells, parathyroid cells and heart (Table I). Presumably, all these effects are mediated through α_2-receptors and involve inhibition of adenylate cyclase. Some physiological changes can be ascribed to the decrease in cAMP induced by α-agonists in these tissues e.g. inhibition of lipolysis, inhibition of insulin secretion and lightening of skin.

α_2-Adrenergic receptors have been identified by radioligand binding studies in other tissues besides platelets, viz. brain, salivary gland, liver, kidney, uterus and adipose tissue (Table I)[1]. In brain and liver the presence of both α_1- and α_2-receptors gave rise to the initial separation of the α-receptors into two classes with different affinities for agonists and antagonists. The α_2-receptors identified to date in rat liver plasma membranes appear to represent 10–20 per cent of the total α-receptors labelled with [^{3}H]dihydroergocryptine[1]. Some of these α_2-receptors have a very high affinity for epinephrine (K_d, approximately 10 nM), whereas others have a much lower affinity (K_d approximately 1 μM, El-Refai, M. F. and Exton, J. H., unpublished observations). It is possible that these latter receptors mediate the inhibitory effect of epinephrine on liver adenylate cyclase since the half-maximal epinephrine concentration for these effects is 3 μM (Ref. 2). The function of the high affinity sites is unknown.

Receptors of the α_2-type are widely distributed in the brain. The binding of agonists to cortical α_2-receptors is decreased by guanine nucleotides and the inhibition is reversed by Mn^{2+}, Mg^{2+} and Ca^{2+}. This is because the cortex contains both high- and low-affinity α_2 binding sites, and guanine nucleotides decrease the number of high-affinity sites, whereas the divalent cations increase the number of these sites[5]. The guanine nucleotides and ions have only minimal effects on the low-affinity binding[5]. In contrast to the divalent cations, Na^+ decreases both high- and low-affinity binding[5] as noted for rabbit platelets[3]. It is not known which cell type(s) contains the α_2-receptors of the brain, but presumably their activation decreases cAMP and may thus modulate synaptic transmission by altering the phosphorylation state of certain neuronal proteins.

Mechanisms involved in α_1-adrenergic responses in liver. The role of calcium

The mechanisms involved in the responses mediated by α_1-receptors are less well defined than those of α_2-receptors. However, growing evidence indicates that activation of these receptors changes cell calcium fluxes and phosphatidylinositol metabolism with attendant alterations in physiological functions (Table II). The clearest evidence for the involvement of α_1-receptors in cell calcium changes comes from studies in liver. Several groups have shown that α-adrenergic stimulation of isolated rat liver cells or perfused rat livers results in alterations in Ca^{2+} fluxes[6,7]. As will be explored in detail below, these alterations result in a rise in cytosolic Ca^{2+} which is responsible for the effects of α-adrenergic stimulation on a variety of processes[8]. The most clear-cut example is the α-adrenergic activation of hepatic glycogenolysis. This response is due to the conversion of phosphorylase b to a, which occurs without a rise in cAMP or a stable modification of cAMP-dependent protein kinase or of phosphorylase b kinase[6,7]. The evidence that it involves Ca^{2+} comes from studies with the chelator EGTA, the divalent cation ionophore A23187, and vasopressin and angiotensin II which produce alterations in hepatocyte Ca^{2+} fluxes similar to those induced by α-agonists[6,7]. In addition, phosphorylase b kinase, the enzyme which converts phosphorylase b to a is allosterically stimulated by concentrations of Ca^{2+} within the range (10^{-8} M to -10^{-6} M) probably occurring in liver cytosol. Further evidence for the involvement of phosphorylase b kinase in α-adrenergic activation of phosphorylase comes from studies with mutant rats lacking this enzyme. Hepatocytes from these rats do not show phosphorylase activation in response to α-agonists, vasopressin or A23187 (Blackmore, P. F. and Exton, J. H. (1981) *Biochem. J.* 198, 379–383).

There is evidence that some other α-adrenergic responses in the liver are Ca^{2+}-dependent. These include the inactivation of glycogen synthase, the stimulation of gluconeogenesis and inactivation of pyruvate kinase, the increase in K^+ fluxes across the plasma membrane, the stimulation of respiration, and the increase in amino acid transport. Evidence is also accumulating showing that many of the enzyme changes induced by α_1-receptor stimulation in liver are due to phosphorylation. For example, incubation of hepatocytes with α-agonists, vasopressin, angiotensin II and the cationophore A23187 leads to increased incorporation of [^{32}P]P$_i$ into phosphorylase, glycogen synthase and pyruvate kinase. It may be hypothesized that many of the α-adrenergic responses in tissues result from the stimulation of a Ca^{2+}-calmodulin protein kinase(s), but evidence for this is very limited at present.

TABLE II. Tissues in which α_1-receptors have been identified and related to Ca^{2+} and phosphatidylinositol changes

Tissue	α_1-Receptors identified by radioligand binding	Role for Ca^{2+} in α-responses indicated	Role for phosphatidylinositol in α-responses indicated
Liver	+	+	+
Salivary	+	+	+
Adipose	+	+	+
Heart	+	−	−
Smooth Muscle	+	+	+
Lacrimal	−	+	+
Brain	+	+	+
Pineal	−	+	+

Several groups have shown that the receptors mediating the effects of α-agonists on rat liver phosphorylase are of the α_1-type[1,6]. Binding studies with [^{3}H]epinephrine and [^{3}H]dihydroergocryptine have identified α_1-receptors in rat liver plasma membranes with high and low affinities for epinephrine[9]. The high affinity α_1-receptors (K_d for epinephrine, about 50 nM) exhibit affinities for α-antagonists and agonists which are extremely close to those found for the effects of these agents on phosphorylase activation and Ca^{2+}-efflux in isolated hepatocytes[9]. It is therefore very likely that they represent the physiological α_1-receptors. As noted above, rat liver plasma membranes also contain α_2-receptors with high affinity for epinephrine (K_d, about 10 nM). The presence of both α_1- and α_2-receptors for epinephrine in the liver has given rise to confusion about the physiologically relevant receptors in liver[1]. This has been caused by the use in one report of a low concentration (10 nM) of [^{3}H]epinephrine to study binding to membranes and of a higher concentration (100 nM) to examine the physiological responses in hepatocytes[2]. In such binding studies, the ligand will bind predominantly to the high affinity α_2-receptors[1], whereas when it is used at physiologically effective concentrations (50–100 nM) it will interact mainly with the high affinity, physiologically relevant α_1-receptors[9]. This illustrates the potential for error when different concentrations of an agonist are used to explore receptors in membranes and physiological responses in cells[1].

The mechanism(s) by which α-adrenergic stimulation raises cytosolic Ca^{2+} in liver is not well understood and some features are in dispute. Two main schemes have been proposed, viz. stimulation of Ca^{2+} influx from the extracellular environment, and mobilization of Ca^{2+} from intracellular stores. It appears that if an influx component contributes to the rise in cytosolic Ca^{2+} in addition to intracellular Ca^{2+} release, it is probably without mechanistic significance. This is because the rapid removal of free Ca^{2+} from the external medium with EGTA does not diminish the stimulation of phosphorylase by α-agonists in hepatocytes[6].

Several investigators have employed measurements of chemical calcium to demonstrate that mitochondria are the major intracellular source from which Ca^{2+} is mobilized by α-adrenergic stimulation in liver (Fig. 2)[6,8,10]. On the other hand, other investigators using ^{45}Ca to label the mitochondrial Ca pool have claimed that α-adrenergic stimulation increases mitochondrial Ca^{2+} uptake, and have suggested therefore that other, unidentified, cellular stores are mobilized. Since the fraction of total cell Ca released during α-stimulation is very large, it is clear that a major intracellular Ca pool must be affected. Efforts to demonstrate the release of Ca^{2+} from other intracellular sites during hormone stimulation of liver have not yielded clear cut results. For example, both decreases and increases in the Ca content of microsomes have been reported[6,8]. Although plasma membranes are known to contain large amounts of calcium, we have been unable to demonstrate any significant change in Ca^{2+} content or ^{45}Ca binding in liver plasma membranes treated with epinephrine (Prpić, V. and Exton, J. H., unpublished observations).

The possibility that intracellular organelles respond to α-agonists directly is unlikely since neither mitochondria nor microsomes possess the appropriate catecholamine receptors[9], and no changes in Ca^{2+} fluxes are seen when epinephrine is added directly to these organelles (Blackmore, P. F., Dehaye, J.-P. and Prpić, V., unpublished observations). Epinephrine is also extensively metabolized following uptake by liver cells and it has been reported that when epinephrine is linked stably to a large molecular weight copolypeptide such that it can only interact with cell-surface receptors, it can still produce all the α-adrenergic actions of free epinephrine[6]. These considerations lead to the conclusion that the intracellular effects of α-agonists are due to a putative signal generated at the plasma membrane. Based on the time course of the cell Ca^{2+} fluxes induced by these agonists, such a messenger must be formed or released within seconds and then inactivated or reaccumulated. Very many factors are known to influence intracellular Ca^{2+} movements, but, to date, none of these factors has been clearly implicated in α-adrenergic phenomena.

The possible role of phosphatidylinositol turnover

Incubation of rat hepatocytes with α_1-agonists, vasopressin and angiotensin II increases the incorporation of [^{32}P]P$_i$ into phosphatidylinositol[11,12]. This response is also seen in many other tissues treated with α-adrenergic, muscarinic cholinergic, or certain other agents which produce cAMP-independent effects[13,14]. The primary event is believed to be phosphatidylinositol breakdown[11–14], which is thought to produce a rise in 1,2-diacylglycerol leading to enhanced resynthesis of the phospholipid. The cellular sites at which these changes occur are uncertain, although it is likely that resynthesis mainly involves the endoplasmic reticulum which is the location of CDP-diacylglycerol:inositol phosphatidyltransferase. The phosphatidylinositol-specific phospholipase C which catalyses phosphatidylinositol breakdown has been found in the cytosol, but it is uncertain whether it is also membrane-bound. The soluble enzyme apparently does not readily attack the phosphatidylinositol of cell membranes, but its action can be stimulated by phosphatidic acid and certain lysophosphatidic acids, and inhibited by phosphatidylcholine and certain lysophosphatidylcholines. Thus, changes in phosphatidylcholine or phosphatidic acid could influence the breakdown of phosphatidylinositol in cell membranes. However, the regulatory significance of these interactions remains to be defined.

Michell[13] has marshalled impressive evidence showing an association between changes in phosphatidylinositol metabolism and cellular Ca^{2+} in many eukaryotic cells exposed to a wide variety of agents. There is considerable evidence that the phosphatidylinositol changes are not secondary to an increase in cytosolic Ca^{2+}, but it is uncertain whether they are primary or parallel events in the alterations in cell Ca^{2+}. The time course of stimulation of [^{32}P]P$_i$ incorporation into phosphatidylinositol in isolated hepatocytes is slower than the release of Ca^{2+} or activation of phosphorylase and requires higher concentrations of agents[11,12]. These data appear to exclude a primary role for phosphatidylinositol synthesis in the Ca^{2+} changes. However, phosphatidylinositol breakdown may occur earlier and it is possible that a very small change in this parameter could result in maximal physiological responses.

Phosphatidylinositol breakdown could increase cytosolic Ca^{2+} by (1) releasing calcium from the plasma membrane; (2) increasing the permeability of the membrane to Ca^{2+} such that there is an influx of extracellular Ca^{2+} and (3) generating an intracellular messenger which causes the release of Ca^{2+} from intracellular organelles[13,14]. However, no clear evidence for any of these mechanisms exists. Initially it was hypothesized that inositol 1,2-cyclic phosphate or inositol 1-phosphate released during phosphatidylinositol breakdown might function as an intracellular messenger. These compounds do not influence Ca^{2+} efflux from mitochondria (Hughes, B. P. and Blackmore, P. F., unpublished observations) and other support for their postulated role is lacking.

Phosphatidic acid has also been proposed as a mediator of muscarinic cholinergic or α-adrenergic effects in smooth muscle and parotid gland[15,16]. This compound is a precursor of phosphatidylinositol and other phospholipids, and may be formed from 1,2-diacylglycerol produced by phosphatidylinositol breakdown. In support of this hypothesis are the observations that phosphatidate accumulates during stimulation of smooth muscle or parotid cells by muscarinic agonists, causes contraction of smooth muscle cells at submicromolar concentration, induces ^{86}Rb efflux from parotid slices, and can act as a Ca ionophore[15,16]. Phosphatidate at 10^{-4}M causes Ca^{2+} release from rat liver mitochondria, but this is due to uncoupling of oxidative phosphorylation (Hughes, B. P., unpublished observations). Another problem with respect to the hypothesis is that the metabolism of phosphatidate is linked to that of other phospholipids and also triacylglycerol. Thus, it seems unlikely that it would be controlled mainly by phosphatidylinositol breakdown, unless the concept of metabolic compartmentation is invoked.

It is logical to expect that phosphatidylinositol breakdown would be linked to the α_1-receptor in the plasma membrane if this were a primary event in the postulated changes in plasma membrane Ca^{2+} binding and permeability. However, the intracellular site of this breakdown is undefined at present.

Nishizuka and associates[17] have put forward an intriguing proposal relating phosphatidylinositol turnover with the activation of a protein kinase dependent on Ca^{2+} and on a phospholipid such as phosphatidylserine. This kinase is present in many tissues and is stimulated by diacylglycerols, especially those containing unsaturated fatty acids. Since phosphatidylinositol breakdown would release such diacylglycerols and is also associated with a rise in cytosolic Ca^{2+}, this group has suggested that the kinase might play a specific role in α-adrenergic and muscarinic cholinergic responses.

α_1-Adrenergic responses in other tissues

Another tissue in which α_1-receptors have been identified and α_1-responses are relatively well-defined is parotid gland[18]. In salivary and also lacrimal glands, α_1 and muscarinic cholinergic agonists increase the permeability of the plasma membrane to K^+ leading to a release of K^+ and an osmotic outflow of water. Two phases of K^+ release can be defined: an initial transient phase which appears to involve the release of Ca^{2+} from an internal source, since it does not depend on extracellular Ca^{2+}, and a second phase which requires the presence of external Ca^{2+} and is therefore thought to involve Ca^{2+} influx[18]. The release of K^+ is associated with increased labelling of phosphatidylinositol, and this is thought to be related to the influx of Ca^{2+}. As noted above, it has been postulated that phosphatidate might link these processes[16].

Insect salivary glands show an increase in K^+ and fluid secretion in response to 5-hydroxytryptamine[14]. In this system, the increased salivary secretion is associated with transepithelial Ca^{2+} transport and phosphatidylinositol breakdown. The effect of 5-hydroxytryptamine on Ca^{2+} transport declines with time, but can be restored by incubating the glands with inositol suggesting that it results from a decrease in phosphatidylinositol concentration[14].

Smooth muscles from most tissues except intestine contract in response to α-adrenergic stimulation, and it is generally accepted that a rise in intracellular Ca^{2+} is involved[19]. Current evidence suggests that contraction is the result of Ca^{2+} stimulation of a calmodulin-dependent myosin light chain kinase. Phosphorylation of the light chains of smooth muscle myosin is necessary for the interaction of this protein with actin to cause contraction.

Smooth muscles may exhibit phasic or tonic contractile responses to α-agonists. The phasic response appears to involve Ca^{2+} mobilization from intracellular sources such as sarcoplasmic reticulum, mitochondria or Ca^{2+} bound to the inner surface of the plasma membrane, whereas the tonic response requires extracellular Ca^{2+}. Phosphatidylinositol turnover is also seen in smooth muscles contracting in response to α-adrenergic, muscarinic cholinergic and H_1 histaminergic agents or 5-hydroxytryptamine, and has been interpreted as being involved in the opening of cell-surface Ca^{2+} gates. In support of this hypothesis, phosphatidate has been reported to cause smooth muscle contraction and to accumulate during cholinergic stimulation[15].

α-Adrenergic stimulation elevates cGMP in vas deferens. This response is also induced by muscarinic cholinergic agents in a Ca^{2+}-dependent manner[20]. It has been proposed that the rise in cGMP is due to an increase in intracellular Ca^{2+} which perhaps activates guanylate cyclase[20]. There is much evidence that the rise in cGMP is not responsible *per se* for the contractile response, but it might function as a negative feedback signal to reduce muscle tone.

Studies of radioligand binding indicate that adipose tissue contains $α_1$- as well as $α_2$-adrenergic receptors and it has been shown that $α_1$-agonists activate phosphorylase and inactivate glycogen synthase in rat adipocytes. These actions may involve Ca^{2+} since they are dependent upon extracellular Ca^{2+} and are mimicked by A23187. Stimulation of fat cells by α-agonists also causes $^{42}K^+$ efflux and increased incorporation of $[^{32}P]P_i$ into phosphatidylinositol.

$α_1$-Receptors are widely distributed in the brain in addition to $α_2$-receptors. As expected, the number of $α_1$-receptors is not decreased by 6-hydroxydopamine treatment which destroys presynaptic membrane components. Further support for a post-synaptic location for these receptors comes from the finding that a series of benzodioxane antagonists show the same specificity toward [^{3}H]WB-4101 binding to α-receptors in brain and peripheral tissues. The function of the $α_1$-receptors of the brain is unknown, but, as in the case of $α_2$-receptors in this tissue, it probably relates to changes in synaptic transmission. There is much evidence that Ca^{2+}, like cAMP, can alter the phosphorylation state of certain neuronal proteins.

There is now abundant evidence that the heart contains α-receptors in addition to the more prevalent β-receptors. Stimulation of the α-receptors produces a positive inotropic, but not chronotropic, response. Studies of radioligand binding to myocardial membranes indicate the presence of both $α_1$- and $α_2$-receptors. The $α_2$-receptors are presumably responsible for the reduction in cAMP and cAMP-dependent protein kinase activity observed in heart when α-agonists are added together with an activator of adenylate cyclase such as isoproterenol. In the absence of such activators, addition of low concentrations of α-agonists results in phosphorylase activation without detectable cAMP accumulation, and it is presumed that this effect is mediated by the $α_1$-receptors and could involve a rise in cytosolic Ca^{2+}.

Concluding remarks

It is clear from radioligand binding and physiological studies that $α_1$- and $α_2$-receptors are separate entities. Although it was initially thought that they differed in their location with respect to adrenergic nerve endings i.e. presynaptic v. post-synaptic, it is now clear that $α_2$-receptors are located at both sites, whereas $α_1$-receptors seem to be exclusively post-synaptic. The presynaptic $α_2$-receptors mediate the feedback inhibition of norepinephrine release from the nerve endings, but the molecular mechanisms are unknown. Activation of the post-synaptic α_2-receptors is associated with a decrease in cAMP to which many of the physiological responses can be attributed. The fall in cAMP is due to inhibition of adenylate cyclase. The inhibition requires GTP and it has been hypothesized that this nucleotide and an inhibitory guanine nucleotide-binding protein are involved in coupling the α_2-receptor to the catalytic component of the cyclase.

Stimulation of α_1-receptors is not associated with changes in cAMP, but results in alterations in cell Ca^{2+}. There may be an influx of extracellular Ca^{2+} through 'gates' in the plasma membrane or a release of Ca^{2+} from intracellular organelles or the plasma membrane. These responses lead to a rise in cytosolic Ca^{2+} and both changes may occur in the same cell. Several possible molecular mechanisms may be suggested, namely, the α_1-receptor may be linked to a Ca^{2+} 'gate' in the plasma membrane or may cause a change in the plasma membrane such that bound Ca^{2+} is released. Alternatively or additionally, activation of the receptor may generate an intracellular messenger at the plasma membrane which then acts on mitochondria and perhaps other organelles to cause Ca^{2+} release.

There is much evidence in a variety of tissues that the activation of α_1-adrenergic, muscarinic cholinergic and certain other receptors is associated with increased turnover of cell phosphatidylinositol. There have been several proposals linking this phospholipid change to alterations in cell Ca^{2+}. Observations with insect salivary glands have provided the strongest evidence for a causal relationship between the two events, but the situation in mammalian tissues is less certain. The hydrolysis of phosphatidylinositol in the plasma membrane could be associated with the opening of a Ca^{2+} 'gate' and the receptors could control the activity of the phospholipase C involved. In addition, the changes in phosphatidylinositol metabolism could lead to the generation of an intracellular second messenger which releases internal Ca^{2+}. There is some evidence in some systems that phosphatidate may fulfil the messenger role, but further work is needed to establish this as a general mechanism.

The natural agonists, epinephrine and norepinephrine, appear to be relatively nonselective in their affinity for α_1- and α_2-receptors. Their α-adrenergic effects on various tissues may therefore be determined mainly by the relative density of α_1- and α_2-receptors. For example, platelets appear to have exclusively α_2-receptors and liver and parotid have mainly α_1-receptors. However, there are some tissues in which both types of receptor are present in approximately equal numbers e.g. uterine muscle, brain and adipose tissue. The presence of the two types of α-receptor in the same tissue has led to considerable confusion in the analysis of receptor binding and metabolic responses in the past. With the emergence of α_1- and α_2-selective antagonists and agonists, the nature and function of these receptors is becoming clearer, but much more work is required to delineate the molecular mechanisms which couple their activation to their various physiological responses.

Reading list

1 Lefkowitz, R. J. and Hoffman, B. B. (1980) *Trends Pharmacol. Sci.* 1, 369–372
2 Jakobs, K. H., Aktories, H. and Schultz, G. (1981) *Adv. Cyclic Nucleotide Res.* 14, 173–187
3 Michel, T., Hoffman, B. B. and Lefkowitz, R. J. (1980) *Nature (London)* 288, 709–711
4 Steer, M. L. and Wood, A. (1979) *J. Biol. Chem.* 254, 10791–10797
5 Rouot, B. M., U'Prichard, D. C. and Snyder, S. H. (1980) *J. Neurochem.* 34, 374–384
6 Exton, J. H., Blackmore, P. F., El-Refai, M. F., Dehaye, J.-P., Strickland, W. G., Cherrington, A. D., Chan, T. M., Assimacopoulos-Jeannet, F. D. and Chrisman, T. D. (1981) *Adv. Cyclic Nucleotide Res.* 14, 491–505
7 Keppens, S., Vandenheede, J. R. and DeWulf, H. (1977) *Biochim. Biophys. Acta* 496, 448–457
8 Murphy, E., Coll, K., Rich, T. L. and Williamson, J. R. (1980) *J. Biol. Chem.* 255, 6600–6608

9 El-Refai, M. F., Blackmore, P. F. and Exton, J. H. (1979) *J. Biol. Chem.* 254, 4375–4386
10 Babcock. D. F., Chen, J.-L. J., Yip, B. P. and Lardy, H. A. (1979) *J. Biol. Chem.* 254, 8117–8120
11 Billah, M. M. and Michell, R. H. (1979) *Biochem. J.* 182, 661–668
12 Kirk, C. J., Michell, R. H. and Hems, D. A. (1981) *Biochem. J.* 194, 155–165
13 Michell, R. H. (1979) *Trends Biochem. Sci.* 4, 128–131
14 Berridge, M. J. (1980) *Trends Pharmacol. Sci.* 1, 419–424
15 Salmon, D. M. and Honeyman, T. W. (1980) *Nature (London)* 284, 344–345
16 Putney, J. W., Jr., Weiss, S. J., Van De Walle, C. M. and Haddas, R. A. (1980) *Nature (London)* 284, 345–347
17 Kishimoto, A., Takai, Y., Mori, T., Kikkawa, U. and Nishizuka, Y. (1980) *J. Biol. Chem.* 255, 2273–2276
18 Putney, J. W., Jr. (1979) *Pharmacol. Rev.* 30, 209–245
19 Bolton, T. B. (1979) *Physiol. Rev.* 59, 606–718
20 Schultz, G., Hardman, J. G., Schultz, K., Baird, C. E. and Sutherland, E. W. (1973) *Proc. Natl Acad. Sci. U.S.A.* 70, 3889–3893

The puzzling 'cascade' of multiple receptors for dopamine
An appraisal of the current situation

A. R. Cools

Department of Pharmacology, University of Nijmegen, P.O. Box 9101, 6500 HB Nijmegen, The Netherlands.

Considering the great variety of criteria that are used to characterize and subdivide dopamine (DA) receptors into distinct sets of two or more subclasses, the main question is how to integrate the available data into one unifying concept. The speculative hypothesis is put forward that we are dealing with a single macromolecular complex of which the conformational mobility varies according to the presence or absence of co-operatively linked serotonergic or noradrenergic subunits, or both, thereby allowing us to discern three biochemically, pharmacologically and functionally distinct DA receptors: DAe, DAi and DAi/e receptors. The vast majority of DA-specific biological responses appear to result from changes in a single subclass of DA receptors: a small number, however, appear to rely on changes in two, or even all three, subclasses of DA receptors. Although the concept as such has not yet evolved into concrete reality, it allows us to prove whether the present-day arguments are fiction or fact.

Since dopamine (DA) has been recognized as a physiologically occurring substance that transmits chemical-bound, stimulus energy from neurons towards target membranes, cells, tissues, organs and other biological entities, it has become evident that it can elicit two functionally opposite effects in otherwise analogous biological systems[1-4]. (1) It increases or decreases the responsiveness of cellular membranes (neurons). (2) It depolarizes or hyperpolarizes cellular membranes (neurons). (3) It increases or decreases the adenylyl cyclase activity (neuronal elements). (4) It increases or decreases the impulse flow (neurons). (5) It increases or decreases the release of neurotransmitters (neurons). (6) It increases or decreases the release of hormones such as prolactin (neuroendocrine cells). (7) It produces vasodilatation or vasoconstriction (blood vessels). Normally, the mentioned biological responses trigger a characteristic sequence of events at hierarchically superior levels of the organization of the organism; accordingly, it is not surprising that the organism, efficiently functioning as a whole in which the individual parts are integrated, also responds in two opposite ways; for instance, DA increases or decreases locomotor activity depending on the target area selected. Analogous to the concept of the alpha- and beta-adrenergic receptors that arose out of the ability to subdivide the adrenergic responses into distinct functional components, the concept of two distinct DA receptors emerged: the excitation-mediating DA receptors and inhibition-mediating DA receptors (DAe and DAi receptors respectively)[1]. The concept itself is elaborated elsewhere in detail[5]. In that concept as well as in the discussion to follow, DA receptors are assumed to be specialized, macromolecular complexes at the outside of the target unit through which DA compounds act to evoke a characteristic biological response. By definition, DA agonists are compounds that interact with DA receptors and are capable of eliciting a maximal biological response, whereas DA antagonists are compounds that interact with DA receptors, but block agonist-induced biological responses either, (a) by chemically altering the receptors or (b) by simple occupancy of the receptors thereby preventing access to the receptors by agonists. Partial DA agonists are compounds that interact with the DA receptors eliciting a biological response that is submaximal regardless of the concentration of partial agonist employed.

Characterization of the above-mentioned biological responses in terms of pharmacological specificity forms the basis for the notion that there are even three subclasses of DA receptors. Considering the pharmacological features of apomorphine, for instance, it turns out that this agent acts like (a) a full agonist in systems in which butyrophenones, but not phenothiazines or benzamides, are the most potent antagonists (vasodilatation in femoral vasculature, climbing in mice, etc.), (b) a partial agonist in systems in which phenothiazines, but not butyrophenones or benzamides, are the most potent antagonists (excitation of snail neurons, etc.), and (c) a potent antagonist in systems in which benzamides, but not butyrophenones, are the most potent antagonists (vasodilatation in renal vasculature, etc.). In fact, each of the three distinct DA receptors is delineated in terms of selective agonists and antagonists (see also below).

In attempts to increase the knowledge about the nature of DA receptors, two new lines of research have recently been introduced: the study of the potency of DA agents to increase the formation of cyclic AMP by activation of intracellular adenylyl cyclase in target cells equipped with DA receptors, and the study of the binding of DA agents to putative DA receptors. The former studies have revealed that some DA target tissues (neostriatum, retina, substantia nigra, bovine parathyroid, etc.) contain specific DA-sensitive adenylyl cyclase; by contrast, other DA target tissues (mammotroph of anterior pituitary, etc.) lack this specific DA-sensitive enzyme. Because of these findings, two subclasses of DA receptors have been postulated[6]: a homogeneous class of DA receptors which are linked to this enzyme (D1 receptors) and a class of DA receptors which are not linked to this enzyme (D2 receptors). As the latter class is solely defined in negative terms, such a dichotomous division is misleading because it neglects the possibility of an additional heterogeneity within that class, and because it excludes the possibility of comparing the pharmacological specificity of the biological events within the same frame of reference. Studies of the binding of DA agents to putative pharmacological receptors are continuously employed to study receptors for endogenous DA. As one of the two basic properties of pharmacological agents, i.e. intrinsic activity (being defined as the maximally attainable biological response that can be elicited by that compound) cannot be assessed in the ligand binding studies, the pattern of relative affinities (potencies) of a series of compounds in interaction with the cellular binding sites is critical to an interpretation of ligand binding data in terms of 'true' DA receptors. Today, there is accumulating evidence in favour of the existence of three subclasses of specific DA binding sites which fulfil many criteria for typifying them as endogenous DA receptors[7]: (a) binding sites with a high affinity for DA agonist and antagonist ligands, (b) binding sites with a high affinity for DA agonist ligands and a low affinity for DA antagonist ligands, and (c) binding sites with a low affinity for DA agonist ligands and a high affinity for DA antagonist ligands.

Considering the great variety of criteria that are used to characterize and subdivide DA receptors into two or more subclasses, the main question is how to integrate the available data into one unifying concept. The speculative hypothesis is put forward that we are dealing with a single macromolecular complex of which the conformational mobility varies according to the presence or absence of co-operatively linked serotonergic or noradrenergic subunits, or both. It will be argued that the receptor-site preferred conformation of DA is threefold; each plays a functional role in the receptors' physiological action.

Actual problems

The DA response process as a rule is built up in three steps, (a) the DA receptor interaction comprising the binding of DA to the macromolecular complexes at the outside of the target unit, (b) the coupling step comprising the biological events which are intermediates between the binding of DA to the cell surface sites and the resulting biological response (e.g. intracellular changes in cyclic AMP formation), and (c) the biological response comprising, (1) transmission of chemical-bound energy from the target unit to other biological entities (release of transmitters such as acetylcholine or glutamate from non-DA neurons equipped with DA receptors and release of hormones such as prolactin from neuroendocrine cells equipped with DA receptors), (2) performance of mechanical work (vasodilatation or vasoconstriction of blood vessels equipped with DA receptors), (3) alteration of the responsiveness of the target unit itself (changes in one or more of the characteristic features of 'presynaptic' or 'autaptic', or both, DA receptors on DA neurons), (4) maintenance of the internal environment of the target unit as well as maintenance of the integrity of its structure (bio-inactivation and storage of DA in DA neurons equipped with 'presynaptic' DA receptors), and (5) organization of the individual parts of the organism into an efficiently functioning whole (bio-inactivation of DA in glial cells equipped with DA receptors and bio-inactivation of DA by enzymes comprising DA receptors). Considering these steps, it is evident that our problem of analysing similarities and dissimilarities between distinct 'DA receptors' is at least threefold.

First: do specific DA binding sites show a real correlation with the specific DA-sensitive intermediate biochemical events between binding of DA agents to the cell surface sites and the resulting biological responses? The preliminary answer to this question is simply *no*: none of the DA binding sites that have been studied with the help of radioligands exhibit the pharmacological specificity of the DA-sensitive adenylyl cyclase linked receptor. As compounds such as 2-amino-6,7-dihydroxytetralin(6,7-ADTN) that behave like 'mixed agonists/antagonists' in the binding studies, in which the DA antagonist flupenthixol is used as radioligand behave like full agonists in the adenylyl cyclase assay, this also holds true for the binding sites labelled with this radioligand despite the high correlation coefficient for the flupenthixol binding v. the adenylyl cyclase assay[8]. Later on, we will see that this statement has to be revised, as the criteria used for labelling a compound as 'agonist', 'mixed agonist/antagonist' or 'antagonist' in binding studies might require some revision.

Second: do the specific DA binding sites show a real correlation with any of the DA-specific biological responses. Again, the answer is *no*. The finding that the relative affinities of the binding of a great variety of DA compounds to sites labelled with butyrophenones show a close correlation

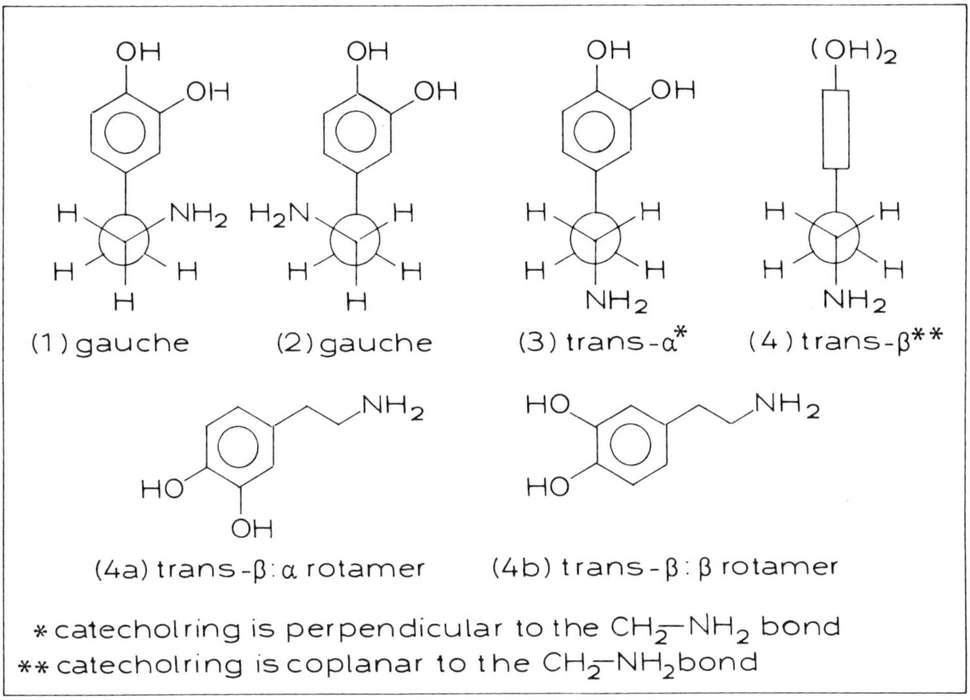

Fig. 1. Outcome of conformational analysis of DA[10].

with the relative potencies of these agents in behavioural tests, in which apomorphine is selected as the tool of choice[9], cannot be taken as evidence. This is because the apomorphine-induced response itself is the combined result of apomorphine-induced activation of one group of DA receptors and apomorphine-induced inhibition of another group of DA receptors (see below); indeed, apomorphine does not behave as a full 'agonist' in the binding assay.

Third: does the specific DA-sensitive intermediate biochemical event between binding of the DA agents to the cellular surface sites and the resulting biological responses show a real correlation with any of the DA-specific biological responses? Again, all researchers agree that the answer is *no*, although the DA-induced excitation of the snail neurons is an exception in this respect (see below).

Given the impossibility of integrating the three distinct steps of the drug-response process because of the apparent lack of real correlations, the only clue left is the structural requirements of the putative DA receptors for the biological activity of DA. As will be discussed below, it is this notion that opens perspectives for understanding the considerable confusion in the field of DA receptor research. The discussion to follow subdivides DA-specific biological responses into, (a) responses elicited by a semi-rigid DA analogue that is allied to the β rotamer of the *trans*-β form of DA, (b) responses elicited by a semi-rigid DA analogue that is more or less allied to the α rotamer of the *trans*-β form of DA, and (c) responses elicited by both DA analogues. This subdivision, which arises out of the fact that DA itself can exist in these forms[10], is chosen in order to facilitate subsequent discussion of the relationships between the pharmacological specificity of, (a) DA-specific biological responses, (b) DA-sensitive adenylyl cyclase, and (c) DA-specific binding sites (Fig. 1).

Potential usefulness of the rigid-analogue approach[10]

Taking advantage of the fact that 2-amino-5,6-dihydroxytetraline (5,6-ADTN) is a semi-rigid DA analogue that corresponds to the α rotamer in contrast to 6,7-ADTN that is closely allied to the β rotamer (Fig. 2), it becomes possible to determine a crucial structural requirement for DA-specific biological responses, which are elicited by 6,7-ADTN, but not by 5,6-ADTN. Subsequent analysis of the relative potencies of DA agents enables further characterization of the DA receptors involved. Finally, comparing the pharmacological specificity of these DA-specific biological responses with that of other DA-specific biological responses, DA-sensitive adenylyl cylase and DA-specific binding sites can help to elucidate the existence of additional features. Having accordingly delineated the features of one group of DA receptors, it becomes possible to characterize the remaining DA-specific biological response by assessing the same principles thereby taking into account the structural requirements for the first class of DA-specific biological responses. The following discussion is not intended to consider all pharmacological features of each group of DA-specific biological responses exhaustively, but simply to focus on a possible explanation for the large number of conflicting data in the literature on DA receptors.

Delineation of DAi receptors

Prototypes of the DA-specific biological responses that are activated by 6,7-ADTN, but not 5,6-ADTN are, the vasodilatation of the renal vasculature[2], accumbens-mediated decrease in the locomotor activity[5], and caudate-mediated ipsilateral turning of the head[5]. The pharmacological specificity of these responses is characterized by the following features: 6,7-ADTN, epinine and, at least in the accumbens and the caudate nucleus, 3,4-dihydroxyphenyl-amino-2-imidazoline (DPI) are full agonists; apomorphine, benzamides, ergot alkaloids and, at least in the accumbens and the caudate nucleus, piribedil are potent and selective antagonists, whereas butyrophenones and phenothiazines are much less specific in this respect. In this context, it should be noted that only *in vitro* studies on the vasculature receptor offer fully reliable data, as the dependent variable in *in vivo* studies also changes as the consequence of DA-induced changes at the ganglionic level (see Refs 2 and 3). Furthermore, it should be noted that the accumbens-mediated locomotor inhibition is only seen in naive, but not nialamide-pretreated, rats[5]. Extrapolating the above-mentioned pharmacological profile to other DA-specific biological responses results in the notion that the hyperpolarization of snail neurons has a similar profile: 6,7-ADTN, epinine and DPI are full agonists; benzamides and ergot alkaloids are potent antagonists, whereas butyrophenones and phenothiazines are much less effective in this respect. Although none of the DA-specific binding sites in vertebrates reveal a profile with the quantitative pharmacological specificity of the mentioned biological responses, attention must be given to the following: (a) 6,7-ADTN, but not apomorphine, behaves like a full 'agonist' in binding studies using spiroperidol as radioligand; (b)

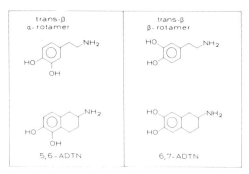

Fig. 2. Correspondence of semi-rigid DA analogues with α and β rotamer forms of trans-β conformation of DA[10].

spiroperidol binding sites consist of a DA and serotonergic (5HT) component; and (c) LSD binding sites in invertebrates reveal not only a profile comparable with that of the mentioned biological responses in the sense that DA, epinine and DPI behave like 'agonists' on the one hand and ergot alkaloids, but not butyrophenones, behave like potent 'antagonists' on the other hand, but also show a high affinity for 5HT compounds. By integrating the available information, the following picture emerges. We are dealing with a DA receptor-site that has a preference for DA agonists existing in the *trans β* rotamer form and, in addition, is closely linked to a 5HT receptor component: 6,7-ADTN, epinine and DPI are full agonists; benzamides, ergot alkaloids, apomorphine and piribedil, but not butyrophenones, are potent antagonists. Apart from the possibility that it is the 5HT component that restricts the DA receptor site preferred conformation of DA, the conformational mobility of the DA receptor site might be such that compounds that exist in the *trans α* rotamer form also have some affinity, thereby acting like non-competitive antagonists of the physiologically active DA receptors. Indeed, compounds such as apomorphine and butyrophenones that primarily interact with DA-specific receptor sites for which agents in the *trans α* rotamer conformation have a high affinity (see below), behave like antagonists in studies on renal vasculature and hyperpolarization of snail neurons. In other words, the macromolecular complex comprising the mentioned DA receptor sites may at least consist of a 5HT component and two DA components, of which only one forms part and parcel of the chain of events that gives rise to the biological response, i.e. the component that accepts agents in the *trans β* rotamer conformation. Although the 5HT component might shift the dynamic equilibrium between the DA component that accepts agents in the *trans α* rotamer conformation towards the physiologically active DA component that accepts agents in the *trans β* rotamer conformation, it must be assumed that there are still some non-physiologically active DA components present, as discussed above. This proposal fits quite well with the well-known suggestion of Josee Leysen that the spiroperidol binding site is 'a unitary receptor complex composed of cooperatively linked subunits for high affinity agonist and antagonist binding, minimally comprised of 2 antagonist sites (5HT and non-physiologically active DA components) and 1 agonist site (physiologically active DA component)'. From now on, it is proposed that the physiologically active DA component should be designated DAi receptors because of the fact that its pharmacological specificity is identical to that of the so-called inhibition-mediating DA receptors in invertebrates and vertebrates.

Delineation of DAe receptors

Keeping the features of the DAi receptors in mind, the question arises whether there are DA-specific biological responses which require DA receptor sites that (a) have a preference for compounds existing in the *trans α* rotamer form (5,6-ADTN; apomorphine), (b) display a pharmacological profile different from that of the DAi receptors, and (c) are not linked to a 5HT component. In this case, there are two DA-specific biological responses that fit into this scheme: caudate-mediated contralateral turning of the head[5], and apomorphine-induced climbing[5]. The pharmacological specificity of these responses can be characterized as follows: apomorphine is a full agonist (5,6-ADTN is not yet tested), butyrophenones, but not benzamides, ergot alkaloids and piribedil, are potent antagonists and DPI lacks any activity, at least in the caudate nucleus. Again, none of the DA-specific binding sites reveal a pharmacological profile comparable with that of the biological responses mentioned. Nevertheless, there are three important sets of data: (a) the affinity of DA for binding sites labelled with the radioligand haloperidol is identical to that of noradrenaline (NE); (b) compounds with a NE component in their spectrum of activity have a relatively high affinity for haloperidol binding sites in contrast to their low affinity for LSD binding sites which are closely allied to the DAi receptors (see above); and (c) haloperidol itself has a relatively high affinity for binding sites labelled with α NE antagonists. These data open the perspective that the DA receptor sites, which have a preference for agents in the *trans* α rotamer conformation, are closely linked to a NE, but not 5HT, component: apomorphine and, probably, 5,6-ADTN are full agonists and butyrophenones, but not benzamides, ergot alkaloids and piribedil, are potent antagonists. In this case too, it might be the NE component that restricts the DA receptor site preferred conformation. Analogous to the DAi receptor, the conformational mobility of this DA receptor site might be such that compounds that exist in the *trans* β rotamer conformation also have some affinity, thereby acting as non-competitive antagonists of the physiologically active DA receptor sites. Indeed benzamides, being potent antagonists of the DAi receptors in physiological studies, behave like weak antagonists in studies on the climbing response in mice. In other words, it is attractive to postulate that the macromolecular complex comprising the latter DA receptor sites may at least consist of a NE component and two DA components, of which only one forms part of the chain of events that gives rise to the biological response, i.e. the component that accepts agents in the *trans* α rotamer conformation. Although the NE component might shift the dynamic equilibrium between the DA component that accepts agents in the *trans* β rotamer conformation towards the physiologically active DA component that accepts agents in the *trans* α rotamer conformation, it must be assumed that there are still some non-physiologically active DA components present as discussed above. From now on, it is proposed to designate the physiologically active DA component as DAe receptors because of the fact that its pharmacological specificity is identical to that of the so-called excitation-mediating DA receptors in vertebrates (note that they differ from those labelled previously as such in snail neurons).

Some remarks on radioligand binding parameters

Regarding the conformational mobility of both DA receptors, it becomes possible to throw new light on the binding data. In the case of the DAe receptors, for instance, it is evident that compounds that primarily interact with DAi receptor sites will shift the equilibrium towards these sites thereby reducing the number of available DAe receptors and, accordingly, inhibiting the amount of specific binding of DAe antagonist ligands to DAe receptor sites. This implies that the order of relative affinities of various DA agents in inhibiting the binding of labelled DAe antagonists does not solely reflect the order of relative potencies of these agents in inhibiting the DAe receptors: it must be an order, in which the relative affinities for DAe and DAi receptor sites are intermingled; indeed, both DAe antagonists, such as butyrophenones and phenothiazines, and DAi antagonists, such as ergot alkaloids and benzamides, are potent displacers of labelled DAe antagonists such as haloperidol[8]. This, together with the fact that apomorphine has a relatively high affinity for the haloperidol binding sites, makes it difficult to substantiate the 'dual agonist/antagonist' concept that assumes that antagonists have a high affinity for DA antagonist binding sites in contrast to agonists that are assumed to have a low affinity for these sites. In fact, differences between affinities for haloperidol binding sites such as those between 6,7-ADTN, that has a low affinity, and apomorphine, that has a relatively high affinity, may simply point to the fact that haloperidol primarily labels DAe receptor sites, although it also, to a lesser degree, labels DAi receptor sites. In this context, it is relevant to note that DAe agonists and antagonists (apomorphine and butyrophenones respectively) as well as DAi agonists and antagonists (6,7-ADTN and ergot alkaloids respectively) have relatively high affinities for binding sites labelled with flupenthixol suggesting that flupenthixol binds to macromolecular complexes comprising DAe and DAi receptor sites in equal amounts. Later on, additional support in favour of this will be mentioned.

Delineation of DAi/e receptors

Having once delineated the characteristic features of the DAi and DAe receptors, the question arises as to whether there are DA-specific responses which require DA receptor sites that show a combined, pharmacological profile. Indeed, there is no doubt that the DA-induced excitation of snail neurons is such a DA-specific biological response: (a) DAi agonists such as 6,7-ADTN and epinine as well as DAe agonists such as apomorphine behave like agonists; in fact, apomorphine being a full agonist of DAe receptors as well as a potent antagonist of DAi receptors behaves as a mixed agonist/antagonist, and (b) both DAi antagonists such as ergot alkaloids and DAe antagonists such as butyrophenones behave as antagonists. Accordingly, it must be assumed that the DA receptor sites under discussion are physiologically active independent of the receptor site preferred conformation of DA. In other words, the macromolecular complex comprising the receptor sites consists of a physiologically active DA component that accepts agents in the *trans* α rotamer form and a physiologically active component that accepts the *trans* β rotamer form; it will be clear that the sites labelled by flupenthixol fulfil all necessary criteria for characterizing them as the DA receptor sites under discussion. The simplest concept to explain the simultaneous occurrence of the DAe and DAi receptor sites is the 'dynamic equilibrium concept', supposing the occurrence of an equilibrium between the DAe and DAi receptor sites thereby assuming that each receptor site similarly contributes to the biological response: absence of the co-operatively linked 5HT as well as NE components might account for such a conformational mobility quite well. From now on, we designate these DA receptor sites as DAi/e receptors. Comparing the relative potencies of specific DAe antagonists for DAe receptors with those of specific DAi antagonists for DAi receptors in physiological tests, it appears that certain DAi antagonists (e.g. benzamides, but not ergot alkaloids) have very low affinities for DAi/e receptors. This explains why the relative affinities of DAe and DAi agents in competing for flupenthixol binding differ so strongly from those predicted on the basis of biological tests, in which just a single subclass of DA receptors is studied. Anyhow, it is possible to delineate the pharmacological properties of the DAi/e receptors as follows: 6,7-ADTN, DPI, epinine and, to a lesser degree, 5,6-ADTN are agonists; apomorphine is a mixed agonist/antagonist; and ergot alkaloids and butyrophenones are potent antagonists in contrast to benzamides which are relatively weak antagonists.

Some remarks on DA-specific cyclic AMP assays

As the pharmacological specificity of the DAi/e receptors fully parallels that of the specific DA-sensitive adenylyl cyclase in neostriatal tissues, this biochemical event appears to be the actual intermediate between the binding of DA agents to the DAi/e receptors and the resulting biological response, although the nature of the response itself is not yet known. Regarding the discrepancies between the outcome of the neostriatal, cyclic AMP assay, in which 6,7-ADTN, but not apomorphine and butyrophenones, acts in a highly selective manner and that of neostriatal, behavioural tests, in which apomorphine and butyrophenones, but not 6,7-ADTN, are highly specific, the question arises as to whether the existence of the DAi/e receptors within neostriatal tissue is simply the result of quirks in the cyclic AMP technique. As mentioned, removal of the cooperatively linked 5HT and NE components will alter DAe or DAi receptor sites, or both, into DAi/e receptor sites by taking away the receptor site preferred conformation of DA; accordingly, the actual existence of physiologically active DAe or DAi receptors might simply be masked by this technique. In this context, it is relevant to note that there is no possibility of comparing the relative potencies of DA agents in stimulating cyclic AMP in the retina with those of these agents in changing DA-dependent biological responses of the retina, since such biological tests are simply not available. Accordingly, it is not yet possible to conclude whether or not the occurrence of DAi/e receptors within the retina are also 'artifacts' of the cyclic AMP assay; the absence of any specific sites for labelled butyrophenones such as domperidone, however, suggests that we are dealing with DAi/e rather than DAe and DAi receptors within the retina. The same holds true for the substantia nigra, although the absence of any biological response with the exception of pure biochemical and electrophysiological effects, confronts us with the possibility that these receptors are 'leftovers', 'silent receptors' or 'acceptors' rather than physiologically active ones.

Apomorphine-induced gnawing, emesis and prolactin response

There are some DA-specific biological responses that show a pharmacological profile that differs from the above-mentioned profiles of DAi, DAe and DAi/e receptors. As theoretical studies exclude the possibility that there are DA receptor sites preferring compounds in a form different from the ones mentioned[10], there is only one explanation left: simultaneous involvement of more than one of the DA receptors delineated above. Indeed, there is hard evidence that the apomorphine-induced gnawing response requires both stimulation of DAe receptors within the neostriatum and inhibition of the DAi receptors within the nucleus accumbens[5]: (a) apomorphine, but not 6,7-ADTN, DPI or epinine, produces gnawing indicating the involvement of DAe receptors; indeed, DAe antagonists such as butyrophenones and phenothiazines are potent inhibitors of this biological response, (b) DAi agonists such as DPI inhibit the gnawing effect suggesting the involvement of DAi receptors; indeed, DAi antagonists such as ergot alkaloids are able to potentiate apomorphine-induced gnawing, and (c) functional as well as topographical differences between the effectiveness of DAe and DAi agonists on the one hand as well as those between the effectiveness of DAe and DAi antagonists on the other hand exclude the involvement of DAi/e receptors in this behavioural test. It is the simultaneous involvement of DAe and DAi receptors in the apomorphine-induced gnawing that explains why the relative affinities of DA agents in competing for haloperidol binding correlate highly with the relative potencies of these agents in inhibiting apomorphine-induced stereotypy[9]; in both cases, we are dealing with an order of potencies, in which the relative affinities for DAe and DAi receptors are fully intermingled.

Apart from the apomorphine-induced gnawing response, there are two additional DA-dependent biological responses that show peculiar, pharmacological profiles that *per se* are highly comparable i.e. apomorphine-induced inhibition of prolactin release, and apomorphine-induced emesis. The main characteristics of their pharmacological specificity are as follows: (a) compounds such as apomorphine and 5,6-ADTN are potent agonists indicating the involvement of DAe receptors; indeed, DAe antagonists such as butyrophenones inhibit the apomorphine-induced responses, (b) compounds such as DPI and 6,7-ADTN are agonists indicating the involvement of DAi receptors; indeed, DAi receptors such as benzamides suppress the apomorphine-induced responses, (c) particular DAi antagonists such as ergot alkaloids and piribedil behave like agonists. As the relative affinities of DA antagonists in suppressing prolactin release or emesis are highly correlated with the relative affinities in competing for haloperidol binding to macromolecular complexes comprising DAe and DAi receptors, as we have discussed above, it must be assumed that both DAe and DAi receptors are involved, thereby similarily contributing to the biological responses under discussion. The recent finding that DA can also stimulate prolactin release implies that a third DA receptor is involved. This together with the fact that ergot alkaloids, but not benzamides, are potent inhibitors of the prolactin release forms the basis for the notion that, in this case, DAi/e receptors are also involved. In contrast to benzamides, which are potent antagonists of DAi receptors but relatively weak antagonists of DAi/e receptors, ergot alkaloids are potent antagonists of both DAi and DAi/e receptors indicating that only inhibition of DAi/e receptors underlies the ability of ergot alkaloids to suppress prolactin secretion. Thus, all three DA receptors are involved in the regulation of prolactin: (a) DAe and DAi receptors which similarly contribute to the DA-specific inhibition of prolactin release, and (b) DAi/e receptors which contribute to the DA-specific stimulation of prolactin release. Until now, there is no reason to assume that this does not hold true for the emetic response.

Synopsis

It is argued that we are dealing with a single macromolecular complex of which the conformational mobility varies according to the presence or absence of co-operatively linked 5HT or NE subunits, or both, thereby allowing us to discern three biochemically, pharmacologically and functionally distinct DA receptors: DAe, DAi and DAi/e receptors. Apart from the fact that the vast majority of DA-specific biological responses result from changes in a single subclass of DA receptors, there are some biological responses that rely on changes in two or, even, all the subclasses of DA receptors. The concept presented is of interest in several aspects. First, it illustrates the possibility of integrating the various concepts of multiple DA receptors into one unifying concept, thereby opening new perspectives for the evaluation of data from binding studies, cyclic AMP essays, and combined pharmacological and physiological studies in animals and man. It allows us to prove whether the present-day arguments are fiction or fact, although the receptor concept as such has not yet evolved into concrete reality. Furthermore, it illustrates that great caution must be exercised in drawing conclusions about the receptors involved when this is based on studies in which just 'classic' DA agonists or antagonists are used. Finally, it offers a number of guidelines for future research in the field of DA receptor research including the design of new drugs.

Reading list

1 Cools, A. R. and Van Rossum, J. M. (1976) *Psychopharmacologia* 45, 243–254

2 Goldberg, L. I., Volkman, P. H. and Kohli, J. D. (1978) *Annu. Rev. Pharmacol. Toxicol.* 18, 57–79
3 Struyker Boudier, H. A. J. (1975) *Catecholamine Receptors in Nervous Tissue*. Ph.D. Thesis, Stichting Studentenpers, Nijmegen
4 Van Rooyen, J. M. (1980) *Drugs and the Mesotelencephalic System*. Ph.D. Thesis, University of Potchefstroom, S.A.
5 Cools, A. R. and Van Rossum, J. M. (1980) *Life Sci.* 27, 1237–1253
6 Kebabian, J. W. and Calne, D. B. (1979) *Nature (London)* 377, 93–96
7 Creese, I. and Sibley, D. R. (1979) *Comm. Psychopharmacol.* 3, 385–395
8 Hyttel, J. (1980) *Psychopharmacology* 67, 107–109
9 Creese, I., Burt, D. R. and Snyder, S. H. (1976) *Science* 192, 481–483
10 Horn, A. S. and Rodgers, J. R. (1980) *J. Pharm. Pharmacol.* 32, 521–524

Multiple dopamine receptors – new vistas

Philip M. Beart

University of Melbourne, Clinical Pharmacology and Therapeutics Unit, Austin Hospital, Heidelberg, Victoria 3084, Australia.

A large body of experimental evidence has revealed the presence of receptor subtypes for acetylcholine, noradrenaline, dopamine, 5-hydroxytryptamine, histamine, GABA and glutamic acid in the CNS. Multiple receptors probably allow differential responses to the same modulator in such a way that the regulation of intra- and inter-neuronal communication can be subjected to subtle and diverse control, and thus their widespread existence is not surprising. A gamut of evidence supporting multiple dopamine receptors has been gathered from model systems such as the renal vasculature, parathyroid gland, rabbit ear artery, mammotrophs of the anterior pituitary, and from studies of emesis[1]. Although the rational classification of these dopamine receptors into subtypes may be possible, the intricacies of the CNS are another matter. This article aims to present some of the new developments relevant to arguments for dopamine receptor subtypes. Readers are referred to recent editions of *TIPS* for articles pertinent to dopamine receptor multiplicity[2,3,4].

Background

Historically, behavioural observations allowed dopamine receptors to be classified as DA-1 and DA-2, and DA_e and DA_i because differential mechanisms were associated with the behaviour elicited by intrastriatal injection of dopaminergic agonists and antagonists[5]. Neither of these receptor classifications has received wide acceptance perhaps because that of Costall and Naylor (DA-1 and DA-2) is 'too behavioural', while that of Cools (DA_e and DA_i) is probably too complex and all-encompassing to be workable. The latter classification certainly needs to be re-analysed with a broader range of agonists and antagonists, but is relevant to motor abnormalities in man and their treatment with antidyskinetic drugs. The nomenclature designating dopamine receptors as D-1 and D-2 was first proposed by Spano and has gained wide acceptance[6]. In this classification, the D-1 receptors was linked to the dopamine-stimulated adenylate cyclase, while the D-2 receptor was not[1]. This criterion has recently been revised for the D-2 receptor to include a decreased responsiveness to synthesize cyclic AMP in response to β-adrenergic agonists[4]. Probably the most significant contribution of studies of the dopamine-stimulated adenylate cyclase has been that not all dopaminergic agonists and antagonists mediate their effect via sites linked to this enzyme. Pharmacologically, dopaminergic ergots (e.g. bromocryptine, lisuride) are high affinity agonists at D-2 receptors and low affinity antagonists at D-1 sites, while (–)-sulpiride is considered to be a selective antagonist for D-2 receptors. Selective antagonists do not exist for D-1 receptors.

Recent articles have questioned the validity of defining receptors by their linkage to adenylate cyclase on the grounds that receptor subtypes should be differentiated purely on their pharmacological characteristics as defined by an extensive series of agonists and antagonists[5], and that there is a paucity of evidence demonstrating a physiological role for cyclic AMP[3]. Peripheral dopamine receptors have been advocated as model systems for central D-1 and D-2 receptors, but complications have arisen even in the renal vasculature and anterior pituitary, which have been put forward as prototypes for D-1 and D-2 receptors respectively. In particular, sulpiride is the most potent antagonist at the dopamine vascular receptor[7], while dopamine-stimulated adenylate cyclase activity has been detected in both anterior and posterior parts of the pituitary gland[8]. Moreover, recent binding studies have suggested the existence of D-3 receptors, apparently not linked to adenylate cyclase, but exhibiting different pharmacological properties to 'classical' D-2 sites[9] (see below). The hypothesis of D-1 and D-2 receptors can currently be regarded as 'under siege', or perhaps more appropriately in need of updating. As a classification it is probably too general, and the dopamine-stimulated adenylate cyclase might be viewed as just one criterion for qualifying a subtype of dopamine receptors.

Radioligand binding assays

A large number of ligands has been employed to study dopamine receptors (Table I), and the massive literature could best be described as confusing. In fact a recent review[5] has suggested that the data when considered together could suggest the existence of 'a haloperidol dopamine receptor, a flupenthixol dopamine receptor and a benzamide dopamine receptor'. However, radioligand binding assays can provide novel insights into receptor multiplicity, but careful attention needs to be given to ligand concentrations, media composition, membrane preparation and the interpretation of binding data. Conclusions about multiple binding sites should not be made

TABLE I. ^{3}H-Labelled ligands employed to study dopamine receptors

Antagonists	Agonists
Haloperidol	Dopamine
Spiroperidol	Apomorphine
Domperidone	N-n-propylnorapo-morphine
Pimozide	ADTN [a]
Sulpiride	Lisuride
Tiapride	Pergolide
Clozapine	Dihydroergocryptine (?)
Cis-flupenthixol	LSD (?)
Cis-piflutixol	

[a]ADTN, 6,7-dihydroxy-2-aminotetralin

from equilibrium studies and Scatchard analyses alone, but need to be supported by the results of dissociation and thermal inactivation experiments. Of course the presence of multiple binding sites for a ligand does not necessarily mean multiplicity of receptors and the functional importance of new 'putative receptors' should be established by traditional pharmacological approaches (e.g. electrophysiological and behavioural experiments).

Observations that dopaminergic agonists were weak displacers of antagonist binding and gave shallow dose–response curves have been interpreted as either interconvertible or distinct agonist and antagonist binding sites. The findings of Nahorski and co-workers may shed light on the situation in that they find by using a wide range of ligand concentrations, with special attention to picomolar concentrations, saturation data consistent with multiple binding sites for [^{3}H]spiperone in the rat corpus striatum[10]. Dopaminergic agonists were potent, selective displacers of binding (IC_{50}s 10–30 nM) to the high affinity site (apparent K_D ca. 30 pM), and sulpiride was surprisingly effective (IC_{50} 40 nM). Whilst inconsistent with behavioural evidence[11], the potency of sulpiride correlates with evidence that [^{3}H]sulpiride binding is potently inhibited by 'classical' neuroleptic drugs, including butyrophenones[12]. The high affinity binding site labelled by [³H]spiperone in striatal membranes may represent a dopamine receptor, but the identity of the low affinity sites, many of which have an affinity in the nanomolar range is unknown. They might represent pharmacologically insignificant sites of a non-specific nature or inactive (spare?) receptors which might be converted to high affinity sites by various stimuli (e.g. nerve trauma or drugs). Multiple binding sites also exist for [³H]sulpiride[6] and have been recently reported for [³H]N-n-propylnorapomorphine[13], and with due care to ligand concentrations may be found for many of the ligands in Table I.

Butyrophenones are weak inhibitors of the dopamine-stimulated adenylate cyclase, but are unlikely to be pure D-2 antagonists because striatal lesions which abolish adenylate cyclase activity also reduce [³H]spiperone binding to 50% of control[14]. [³H]-domperidone is the 'in vogue' butyrophenone, having greater specificity than spiperone[9]. [³H]cis-flupenthixol may be a useful ligand for studying adenylate cyclase-linked dopamine receptors since the order of potency of neuroleptic drugs in inhibiting its binding to rat striatal membranes is similar to that observed for the inhibition of the cyclase[15]. Haloperidol and spiroperidol displaced [³H]cis-flupenthixol in a biphasic manner, and the butyrophenones were suggested to bind to both high and low affinity sites (but preferentially to the latter). These sites represented 20 and 80% respectively of specific [³H]cis-flupenthixol binding for which saturation analysis showed a single population of binding sites. Perhaps the key finding of these binding experiments was that sulpiride, domperidone, molindone and metoclopramide (postulated specific D-2 antagonists) were much weaker displacers of [³H]cis-flupenthixol binding (IC$_{50}$s 6–60 μM) than previously noted for [³H]spiperone.

Ergots, which may be specific D-2 agonists, were very weak inhibitors of [³H]cis-flupenthixol binding, but potent displacers of [³H]spiperone binding. The striatal binding sites labelled by [³H]cis-flupenthixol are both pharmacologically and anatomically distinct from those labelled by [³H]spiperone[14].

Biphasic displacement curves found with [³H]domperidone and [³H]apomorphine and a small range of dopaminergic agonists and antagonists have been used to propose two new receptors, D-3 and D-4[9]. Thermal inactivation studies provided further support for the new sites, but the evidence must be regarded as preliminary. Nevertheless, D-3 receptors are believed to represent in part autoreceptors on striatal dopaminergic nerve terminals, while D-4 receptors seem to be localized partly on intrastriatal neurones: both have also been found in the nucleus accumbens and olfactory tubercle. Laduron has recently suggested that the postulated existence of subtypes is 'probably a short-lived fashion', and that a unitary concept with subunits of a receptor complex is the most plausible hypothesis[3].

Multiple dopamine receptors – the future

Obviously the classification of dopamine receptors as D-1 and D-2 is too general and new hypotheses are required which take into account recent evidence from

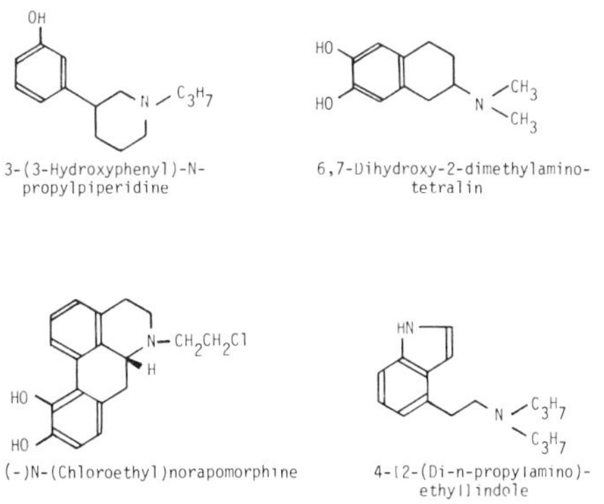

3-(3-Hydroxyphenyl)-N-propylpiperidine

6,7-Dihydroxy-2-dimethylamino-tetralin

(−)N-(Chloroethyl)norapomorphine

4-[2-(Di-n-propylamino)-ethyl]indole

Fig. 1.

radioligand binding studies. These have to be considered with great caution as most are carried out in homogenates containing very heterogenous populations of receptors with ligands of questionable specificity. Radioligand binding has much to offer, but it is in its infancy, and the currently-available dopaminergic ligands should be regarded as just the forerunners: recent pharmacological evidence suggests that a new battery of ligands is just around the corner. The presently-available neuroleptic drugs are unlikely to reveal new vistas as they lack specificity and are incredibly subject to surface phenomena – certainly novel classes of neuroleptic drugs are needed.

New agonist ligands may offer light at the end of the tunnel. 6,7-Dihydroxy-2-dimethylaminotetralin[16] (TL-99) and 3 - (3 - hydroxyphenyl) - N - propylpiperidine[17] (3-PPP, Fig. 1) are two such agonists with selectivity for autoreceptors on axonal nerve terminals, and their specific actions indicate that molecules can be designed with selectivity for receptor subtypes. Dopaminergic ergots at first sight look unsuitable as they possess too much affinity for noradrenergic and serotonergic sites. Perhaps simple indoles related to that synthesized by Cannon and his group (Fig. 1), and proposed as the pharmacophore for these ergots will offer a clue in this direction[18]. The recently available aporphine, $(-)N$ - (chloroethyl) norapomorphine (Fig. 1), offers the possibility of irreversibly labelling receptors for their purification[19]. The phenylbenzazepine, SKF 38393, has been available for a number of years and although possessing interesting and selective pharmacological properties, no attempt appears to have been made to study related analogues.

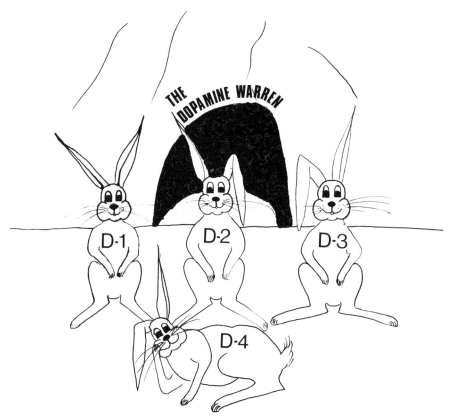

'The trouble with us is that we don't know when to stop.'

Conclusions

The large range of currently-available dopamine agonists has not been exhaustively evaluated in microelectrophoretic studies in any dopaminergic brain region to determine order of potencies or the existence of differential antagonism by classes of neuroleptic drugs. Although many agonists have been studied at peripheral dopamine receptors and in behavioural experiments, specific actions at pre- and post-synaptic receptors in the CNS also need to be fully delineated using either the rotating rodent model or that employing γ-butyrolactone-induced blockade of impulse flow. A comparison should be made to the pharmacology of GABA-mimetics in that over 100 GABA analogues, including at least 50 of restricted conformation, have been tested by microelectrophoresis on central GABA receptors, and most have also been evaluated in isolated preparations. Thus, the potencies of GABA analogues observed in radioligand binding studies can be readily compared with *in-vivo* pharmacological data. Pharmacological screening programmes have much to offer.

The scientific literature pertaining to multiple dopamine receptors is, at best, very confusing and a unifying hypothesis relating functional, anatomical and pharmacological distinctions needs to be developed. How might subtypes of dopamine receptor be classified? Obviously the rank order of potency of a series of agonists would be important. An anatomical criterion would also need to be included (pre- or post-synaptic) and could be determined with specific agonists or with the aid of lesioning techniques. Certainly it is clear that dopamine receptors cannot be classified as excitation- or inhibition-mediating because dopamine released by striatal nerve terminals of the nigrostriatal pathway has an excitatory action, and inhibitory responses are only attributable to recurrent collaterals which drive inhibitory non-dopaminergic interneurones[20]. A hypothesis including differential sensitivities to antagonists would be useful and although 'classical' and 'atypical' neuroleptic drugs have been defined behaviourally[11], it is difficult to see how such a criterion could be included in a classification of receptors. As mentioned above, the dopamine-stimulated adenylate cyclase will need to be considered. The pieces of the jigsaw will not be assembled easily into a workable hypothesis.

Acknowledgements

It is a pleasure to acknowledge discussions with Andrew Gundlach, Bevyn Jarrott, Roger Summers and Jacqui Thomson.

Reading list

1 Kebabian, J. W. and Calne, D. B. (1979) *Nature (London)* 277, 93–96
2 Calne, D. B. (1980) *Trends Pharmacol. Sci.* 1, 412–414
3 Laduron, P. (1980) *Trends Pharmacol. Sci.* 1, 471–474
4 Kebabian, J. W. and Cote, T. E. (1981) *Trends Pharmacol. Sci.* 2, 69–71
5 Costall, B. and Naylor, R. J. (1981) *Life Sci.* 28, 215–229
6 Spano, P. F., Memo, M., Stefanini, E., Fresia, P. and Trabucchi, M. (1980) in *Receptors for Neurotransmitters and Peptide Hormones* (Pepeu, G., Kuhar, M. J. and Enna, S. J., eds), pp. 243–251, Raven Press, New York
7 Goldberg, L. I. (1979) in *The Neurobiology of Dopamine* (Horn, A. S., Korf, J. and Westerink, B. H. C., eds), pp. 541–551, Academic Press, London
8 Ahn, J. S., Gardner, E. and Makman, M. H. (1979) *Eur. J. Pharmacol.* 53, 313–317
9 Sokoloff, P., Martres, M. P. and Schwartz, J. C. (1980) *N.S. Arch. Pharmacol.* 315, 89–102
10 Howlett, D. R. and Nahorski, S. R. (1980) *Life Sci.* 26, 511–517
11 Ljunberg, T. and Ungerstedt, U. (1978) *Psychopharmacologia* 56, 239–247
12 Woodruff, G. N. and Freedman, S. B. (1981) *Neuroscience* 6, 407–410
13 Near, J. A. and Mahler, H. R. (1981) *J. Neurochem.* 36, 1142–1151
14 Leff, S., Adams, L., Hyttel, J. and Creese, I. (1981) *Eur. J. Pharmacol.* 70, 71–75

15 Cross, A. J. and Owen, F. (1980) *Eur. J. Pharmacol.* 65, 341–347
16 Goodale, D. B., Rusterholz, D. B., Long, J. P., Flynn, J. R., Walsh, B., Cannon, J. G. and Lee, T. (1980) *Science* 210, 1141–1143
17 Hjorth, S., Carlsson, A., Wikstrom, H., Lindberg, P., Sanchez, D., Hacksell, U., Arvidsson, L. -E., Svensson, U. and Nilsson, J. L. G. (1981) *Life Sci.* 28, 1225–1238
18 Cannon, J. G., Demopoulos, B. J., Long, J. P., Flynn, J. R. and Sharabi, F. M. (1981) *J. Med. Chem.* 24, 238–240
19 Costall, B., Fortune, D. H., Law, S.-J., Naylor, R. J., Neumeyer, J. L. and Nohria, V. (1980) *Nature (London)* 285, 571–573
20 York, D. H. (1979) in *The Neurobiology of Dopamine* (Horn, A. S., Korf, J. and Westerink, B. H. C., eds), pp. 395–415, Academic Press, London

Is it possible to integrate dopamine receptor terminology?

Johan Offermeier and Johlene M. van Rooyen

Department of Pharmacology and MRC Unit for the Design of Catecholaminergic Drugs (RUDCAD), Potchefstroom University, Potchefstroom 2520, South Africa.

Over the past decade, scientists working in the different fields of dopaminology have found it increasingly difficult to explain clinical and experimental data on the basis of a single type of dopamine (DA)-receptors in the mammalian brain. This has led to the prodigious classification of DA-receptors. These receptors have been designated differently depending upon the individual preferences of scientists and the approaches they used. Consequently some confusion arose in DA-receptor terminology. Certain of these terminologies and the approaches used to arrive at them will be discussed briefly.

Presynaptic DA receptors (autoreceptors)

In 1975 Carlsson suggested that presynaptic DA-receptors, which he designated DA-autoreceptors, may play a role in the receptor-mediated feedback control of DA turnover[1]. This suggestion was based on the observation that the receptor-mediated control of DA synthesis persists after axotomy of central dopaminergic neurons as indicated by inhibition and stimulation of DA synthesis induced by DA-agonists and antagonists respectively. Carlsson[1] also suggested that the paradoxical responses to low doses of DA-agonists, for instance the inhibition of locomotor activity (LA) elicited by low doses of apomorphine, may be mediated via stimulation of DA-autoreceptors.

More recently Anden's group[2] provided evidence which suggests that DA-autoreceptors and post-synaptic DA-receptors are not identical. They investigated the effects of sulpiride and metoclopramide on pre- and post-synaptic DA-receptors in the rat brain on the antagonism of the apomorphine-induced inhibition of DA-synthesis in the absence of nerve impulses and on the blockade of apomorphine-induced rotation following unilateral inactivation of the corpus striatum, respectively. They found that sulpiride was more potent in blocking post- than pre-synaptic receptors while the reverse applied to metoclopramide.

Furthermore, Carlsson's group has synthesized a new DA analogue, N-n-propyl-3-(3-hydroxyphenyl) piperidine (3-PPP), which appears to be a centrally-acting selective DA-autoreceptor agonist which consistently fails to produce signs of post-synaptic DA-receptor activation[3].

D1 (adenylate cyclase-linked) and D2 (non-adenylate cyclase-linked) DA receptors

Although the presence of DA-sensitive adenylate cyclases in virtually all mammalian brain areas innervated by dopaminergic nerve terminals is well documented, the exact physiological role of DA-sensitive adenylate cyclases remains to be elucidated. Evidence for the presence

TABLE I. Pharmacological discrimination between D1- and D2-receptors. (After Kebabian and Calne[4])

	D1-receptors	D2-receptors
Dopamine	Agonist (micromolar conc.)	Agonist (nanomolar conc.)
Apomorphine	Dualist (micromolar conc.)	Agonist (nanomolar conc.)
Bromocriptine	Antagonist (micromolar conc.)	Agonist (nanomolar conc.)
Phenothiazines	Antagonists	Antagonists
Butyrophenones	'Weak' antagonists	'Potent' antagonists
Sulpiride	No effect	Antagonist
Molindone	No effect	Antagonist

of DA-receptors not linked to adenylate cyclases is also well documented. These include the DA-autoreceptors on nigrostriatal neurons, DA-receptors in the pituitary and DA-receptors in the striatum[4]. The nomenclature designating DA-receptors linked to adenylate cyclases as D1, and DA-receptors not linked to adenylate cyclases as D2, is at present widely accepted. Various DA-agonists and DA-antagonists are capable of discriminating between the D1- and D2-receptors, as summarized in Table I.

Pharmacological evidence suggests that the DA-receptor at which dopaminergic transmission is defective in Parkinson's disease is of the D2-type. The D2-agonist bromocriptine, which antagonizes the effect of DA on DA-sensitive adenylate cyclases, is effective in the treatment of Parkinson's disease. The DA-antagonist sulpiride, which has no effect on DA-sensitive adenylate cyclase, can induce Parkinsonian-like side effects in man[4]. Similarly, pharmacological evidence indicates that D2-receptor activation may play a role in the mediation of certain psychotic behaviors; bromocriptine can induce a florid psychosis and sulpiride has antipsychotic effects in man. Crow has also provided evidence for a possible correlation between D2-receptor supersensitivity and the symptomatology of the type 1 syndrome of schizophrenia[5].

³H-neuroleptic and ³H-agonist binding sites

From studies in which the abilities of drugs to displace the specific binding of radio-labeled DA-agonists or DA-antagonists were determined, evidence for the presence of multiple classes of DA binding sites in the mammalian brain has emerged. Assessment of these studies indicates that the mammalian brain contains two types of specific DA binding sites, (a) sites which are preferentially labeled by classical DA-antagonists and (b) sites which are preferentially labeled by classical DA-agonists. Recent evidence indicates that these two types of specific DA binding sites are distinct molecular entities (see Ref. 6).

There is no conclusive evidence that any of the binding sites indentified with the ³H-neuroleptics or ³H-agonists are in any way related to the D1-receptor which regulates adenylate cyclase activity in the striatum, as manifested by the differences in apparent affinities. However, specific binding sites for which the affinity is in the same order of magnitude as the IC_{50} for inhibition of striatal DA-sensitive adenylate cyclase, have been identified for α-cis flupenthixol[7].

The localization of the ³H-neuroleptic and the ³H-agonist binding sites remains controversial. Seeman's group provided arguments (not substantiated by Creese and Snyder[8]) in favour of a presynaptic localization of the ³H-agonist binding sites and a post-synaptic localization of the ³H-neuroleptic binding sites[9]. Seeman furthermore suggested that the ³H-neuroleptics preferentially label post-synaptic

TABLE II. The mechanisms of action of drugs on DAe- and DAi-receptors

	Neostriatal DAe-receptors	Mesolimbic DAi-receptors
Agonists	Apomorphine	DPI
Antagonists	Haloperidol	Piribedil
		Ergometrine

D2-receptors and designated the presynaptic receptors which are preferentially labeled by agonists as 'D3-receptors'[10].

Dopamine excitatory- and dopamine inhibitory-receptors

As early as 1976, Cools and van Rossum provided evidence for the presence of at least two types of DA-receptors involved in behavioral regulation in mammals. These receptors, because of their pharmacological similarity to the DA-receptors mediating excitation and inhibition respectively of *Helix aspersa* neurons, were designated DA excitation-mediating (DAe)- and DA inhibition-mediating (DAi)-receptors[11]. According to the DAe- and DAi-receptor concept certain dopaminergic behaviors, i.e. contralateral turning and LA, depend upon a functional balance between the systems associated with these two types of receptors.

Any shift in the balance in favor of DAe-receptor activation as caused by DAe-agonists or DAi-antagonists (Table II) in the cat caudate nucleus (when unilateral) will induce contralateral head turning whereas a shift in the balance of DAi-receptor activation will induce ipsilateral turning. A shift in the balance in favor of DAe-receptor activation in the rat

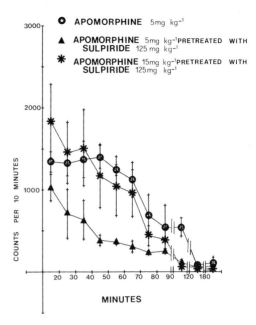

Fig. 1. Antagonism of the effects (mean ± SEM) of intraperitoneal (i.p.) injection of apomorphine (5 mg kg^{-1}) on LA in the rat by the i.p. administration of sulpiride (125 mg kg^{-1}) half an hour before apomorphine. Sulpiride antagonism of apomorphine-induced LA can be completely surmounted by increasing the dose of apomorphine to 15 mg kg^{-1}.

nucleus accumbens (when bilateral) increases LA whereas a shift in favor of DAi-receptor activation decreases LA. Activation of DAi-receptors in the cat caudate as caused by bilateral injections of (3,4-dihydroxyphenylamino)-2-imidazoline (DPI), furthermore, causes facial dyskinesias[11].

Furthermore, Cools and van Rossum suggested that the distribution of these two types of DA-receptors is heterogenous and that the dopaminergic neurons innervating them are distinguishable by internal and biochemical differences. Since 1976, Cools

TABLE III. Internal differentiation of the dopaminergic neurons innervating DAe- and DAi-receptors[6,11]

	DAe-receptor innervating neurons	DAi-receptor innervating neurons
Anatomical origin	A8 and A9 areas of midbrain	A10 area of midbrain
Histochemistry	Diffuse DA fluorescence	Dotted DA fluorescence
Biochemistry	High DA turnover rate	Low DA turnover rate
Post-natal development	Late	Early

TABLE IV.

	Dopamine autoreceptors (presynaptic)	Post-synaptic dopamine receptors	
	? D3	D1 (DAi?)	D2 (DAe?)
Cyclase linked	No	Yes	No
Selective radioligand	[^{3}H]DA	[^{3}H]α-flupentixol	[^{3}H]haloperidol
Selective agonist	PPP	DPI?	bromocriptine, apomorphine
Selective antagonist	metoclopramide	piribedil?[a]	sulpiride

[a] Based upon the apparently competitive antagonism of DA-induced increase of c-AMP in rat NAS homogenates by piribedil (Fig. 3).

and van Rossum have substantiated the original concept of DAe- and DAi-receptors, including the predicted correlation with anatomical, histochemical, biochemical and functional features of distinct neuronal structures in which they occur, as summarized in Table III[6,11].

Integration of the data pertaining to multiple DA-receptors

From the foregoing, it would appear that

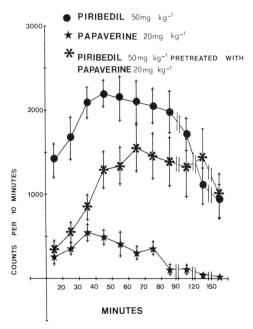

Fig. 2. Antagonism of the effects of piribedil (50 mg kg^{-1}; i.p.) on LA in the rat by the administration of papaverine (20 mg kg^{-1}; i.p.) half an hour before piribedil.

DA-receptors can be divided according to biochemical (adenylate cyclase linkage; ligand binding studies), behavioral and pharmacological criteria. It would also appear that a clear differentiation can be made between presynaptic DA-autoreceptors and post-synaptic DA-receptors (Table IV). Furthermore, a distinction may be made between D1- (cyclase-linked) and D2- (non-cyclase-linked) post-synaptic receptors (Table IV).

It is, however, more difficult to fit Cools and van Rossum's data into this scheme. From the work done in our own laboratory it would appear that the post-synaptic DAe-receptors in the rat nucleus accumbens mediating increases in LA are not cyclase-linked and may therefore be classified as D2-receptors. We demonstrated that sulpiride antagonism of apomorphine-induced locomotor activity (LA) is surmountable by increasing the dose of apomorphine (Fig. 1). This would suggest that apomorphine acts as an agonist on a population of DA-receptors (i.e. not cyclase-linked) on which sulpiride acts as an antagonist.

We have previously shown that piribedil-induced LA, unlike apomorphine-induced LA, is mediated via an antagonistic action on DAi-receptors[12]. We were furthermore able to demonstrate that the phosphodiesterase inhibitor papaverine attenuates piribedil-induced LA (Fig. 2) and that piribedil antagonizes

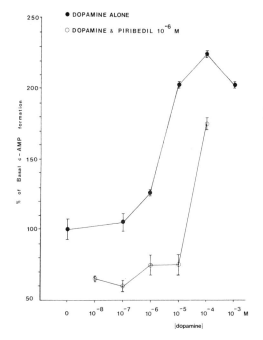

Fig. 3. Antagonism of DA-mediated increases in c-AMP formation in homogenates prepared from the rat NAS by piribedil (10^{-6}M).

DA-induced increases in cyclic adenosine monophosphate (c-AMP) in the rat nucleus accumbens (Fig. 3). These findings would suggest that the DAi-receptor may, in some way, be linked to an adenylate cyclase mechanism and may therefore have certain characteristics in common with the D1-receptor.

Reading list

1 Carlsson, A. (1975) in *Modern Pharmacology-Toxicology: (Pre- and Postsynaptic Receptors)* (Usdin, E. and Bunney, W. E., Jr., eds), Vol. 3, pp. 49–63, Marcel Dekker, Inc., New York
2 Alander, T., Andén, N.-E. and Grabowska-Andén, M. (1980) *Naunyn-Schiedebergs Arch. Pharmakol.* 312, 145–150
3 Hjorth, S., Carlsson, A. and Lindberg, P. (1980) *Psychopharmacol. Bull.* 16, 85–90
4 Kebabian, J. W. and Calne, D. B. (1979) *Nature (London)* 277, 93–96
5 Crow, T. J. (1980) *Br. Med. J.* 280, 66–68
6 Cools, A. R. and van Rossum, J. M. (1980) *Life Sci.* 27, 1237–1253
7 Hyttel, J. (1978) *Life Sci.* 23, 551–556
8 Creese, I. and Snyder, S. H. (1979) *Eur. J. Pharmacol.* 56, 277–281
9 Nagy, J. I., Lee, T., Seeman, P. and Fibiger, H. C. (1978) *Nature (London)* 274, 278–281
10 Titeler, M., List, L. and Seeman, P. (1978) *Commun. Psychopharm.* 3, 411–420
11 Cools, A. R. and van Rossum, J. M. (1976) *Psychopharmacologia* 45, 243–254
12 Offermeier, J. and van Rooyen, J. M. (1979) *Psychologie Med.* 11, 187–204

Dopamine-receptor agonist with apparent selectivity for autoreceptors:
A new principle for antipsychotic action?

J. Lars G. Nilsson and Arvid Carlsson

Faculty of Pharmacy, BMC, University of Uppsala, Box 574, S-751 23 Uppsala, Sweden and Department of Pharmacology, University of Gothenburg, Box 33031, S-400 33 Gothenburg 33, Sweden.

Dopamine in the brain is attracting an ever-increasing interest because of its fundamental role in mental and motor functions and in the pathogenesis of e.g. schizophrenia and Parkinson's disease. This article describes a new principle in the pharmacological manipulation of dopamine.

Dopaminergic neurons and their regulation

Dopamine (DA) is a neurotransmitter in the central and probably also in the peripheral nervous system. In the CNS, DA has often been linked to the pathology of various neurological and psychiatric disorders including Parkinson's disease, schizophrenia, Huntington's chorea and other hyperkinetic conditions. DA is not present uniformly throughout the brain, but is largely localized to specific brain areas, e.g. the striatum and the limbic system. These areas are rich in DA nerve terminals and are therefore considered to be under the control of DA neurons. Abnormal dopaminergic transmission in these areas may consequently contribute to the development of several neuropsychiatric disorders.

As a transmitter, DA is synthesized in the neurons and is released into the synaptic cleft by the nerve impulse, thus eliciting a physiological effect via the post-synaptic receptors. The regulation of the nerve activity such as the impulse flow and the synthesis, release and metabolism of the transmitter is also DA-receptor mediated via a feedback control system. This feedback regulation involves post-synaptic receptors, with neuronal loops transferring information back to the cell body of the presynaptic neuron, and also 'presynaptic' receptors or autoreceptors of the presynaptic neuron. Many drugs used in the treatment of neuropsychiatric disorders have activities which can influence this neuronal regulation system via direct or indirect receptor activation or blockade (for reviews, see Refs 1 and 2).

Dopamine receptors

An important piece of evidence for the

existence of DA-autoreceptors is the so-called 'paradoxical response' to apomorphine. Doses of apomorphine, at least one order of magnitude below that required for producing stereotyped behaviour in the rat, can inhibit the DA synthesis in striatum and in the limbic system in a dose-dependent manner. These low doses also cause an inhibition of locomotor activity, compatible with a reduction in the release of DA. Also, in man, low doses of apomorphine have been shown to exert antipsychotic and antidyskinetic effects[3,4]. This 'paradoxical' effect has been attributed to a selective stimulation of DA autoreceptors at low doses whereas higher doses stimulate e.g. locomotor activity via post-synaptic receptors. This biphasic response also indicates that some structural difference might exist between autoreceptors and post-synaptic DA-receptors. An extensive review of the brain DA-receptors and their agonists and antagonists has recently been published by Seeman[5].

In recent years, the possibility of developing direct DA-receptor agonists with suitable pharmacokinetic properties has attracted increased attention. The advantage of direct post-synaptic receptor agonists to e.g. the precursor L-dopa would be that they act independently of the pre-synaptic neuron. Since several subclasses of DA-receptors are believed to exist, a gain in specificity would be achieved if only one type of receptor could be activated. Higher efficacy might also be obtained, especially under conditions where the pre-synaptic neuron is deficient or has degenerated, as in Parkinson's disease or senile dementia. A disadvantage might be increased risk of overdosage.

All the major antipsychotic drugs used today are receptor-blocking agents, acting mainly on dopamine receptors. However, their usefulness is often limited, which may be partly due to insufficient specificity. An alternative way of achieving anti-dopaminergic activity would be to develop a dopaminergic receptor agonist with selectivity for dopaminergic autoreceptors. Since the autoreceptors are activated already at very low doses of the agonist, it is likely that these receptors have a higher affinity for the agonist and consequently that they could be triggered by compounds that have no affinity for the post-synaptic receptors. Based on these considerations we started the search for compounds with selectivity for the DA autoreceptors.

Screening for DA-receptor agonists with selectivity for autoreceptors

The screening program for compounds with central dopaminergic activity and selectivity for DA-autoreceptors includes inhibition of DA biosynthesis (as evidenced by inhibition of dopa accumulation after inhibition of the aromatic L-amino acid decarboxylase) as a biochemical test and assessment of locomotor activity as a functional test using reserpinized rats. Depending on the observations in these tests, other confirming experiments are performed (for a detailed presentation see Ref. 6).

In the biochemical screening method we use the ability of direct DA-receptor stimulants to reduce the dopa-synthesis rate in the presynaptic neurons. This decreased synthesis is caused by an inhibition of tyrosine hydroxylase mediated via negative feedback systems. The amounts of accumulated dopa in striatum, in the limbic forebrain and in the remaining hemispheral portions of the rat cerebrum (mainly cortex; in this area noradrenaline neurons rather than DA neurons predominate) were determined. Dose–response curves of the test compounds were constructed (s.c. administration) and the dose required to obtain 50% of the maximal dopa-level (ED_{50}) from corresponding control brain portions was estimated.

The biochemical screening method has high sensitivity, measuring effects at very low doses of the DA-receptor stimulants.

At doses equal to the ED_{50} values no behavioural stimulation occurs in reserpine-treated animals. This indicates that no appreciable post-synaptic receptor stimulation occurs at the doses eliciting the biochemically measured effects. Instead the effect is likely to be mediated via the autoreceptors. For behavioural studies, reserpinized rats were given the drug either s.c. or orally, and placed in a motility meter. Increased motility, which could be blocked by haloperidol, was taken as evidence of post-synaptic DA-receptor stimulation. The duration of action, as well as the total number of motor activity counts were determined. Hence the combination of the biochemical and the behavioural test methods makes it possible to distinguish between stimulation of pre- and post-synaptic DA receptors.

3-PPP and its pharmacological profile

In our search for new specific dopamine-receptor agonists we synthesized and tested the DA analogue 3-(3-hydroxyphenyl) - N - n - propylpiperidine (3-PPP) (Fig. 1) and found that it produced all the actions observed after low doses of apomorphine. However, even after nearly lethal doses to rats 3-PPP did not cause any signs of post-synaptic dopaminergic activity. 3-PPP thus seems to act selectively on the dopaminergic autoreceptors. The pharmacological profile of 3-PPP will be illustrated below (for a more detailed description, see Ref. 7).

The most striking behavioural action of 3-PPP in rats and mice is a marked inhibition of exploratory activity (Fig. 2). No stimulatory effects or stereotyped behaviour occur at any dosage, and the action of reserpine is not antagonized (Table I). Biochemically, there is an inhibition of the dopa formation in the dopamine neurons but not in the noradrenaline neurons (reserpine-pretreated animals,

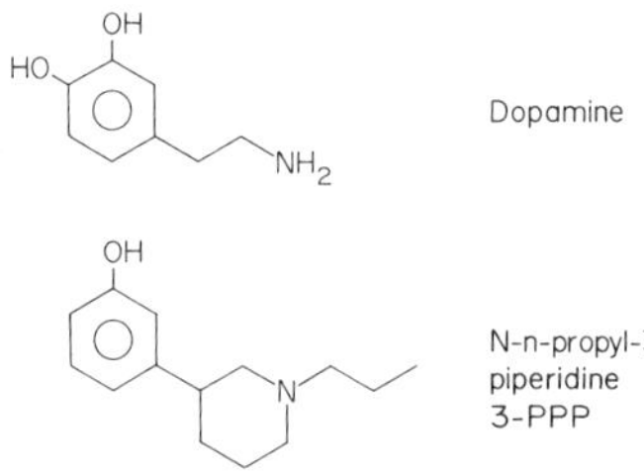

TABLE I. 3-PPP: effects on reserpine-induced hypomotility

Treatment	Rat locomotor activity (counts 90 min^{-1})	N
A. Reserpine + saline	32 ± 11	4
B. Reserpine + 3-PPP	62 ± 7 N.S.	3
C. Reserpine + apomorphine	624 ± 51***	4

Rats were given reserpine (10 mg kg^{-1} i.p.) followed 6 h later by 3-PPP (32 mg kg^{-1} s.c.), apomorphine (1 mg kg^{-1} s.c.) or saline, and their locomotor activity was subsequently recorded (accumulated counts 0–90 min). Shown are the means ± SEM. Statistical significances were calculated by student's t-test. *** $P < 0.001$ and N.S. = not significant, $P > 0.05$ v. reserpine controls (A). (From Hjorth et al. (1980) Psychopharmacol. Bull. 16, 85–90.)

Fig. 1. (a) Dopamine, (b) 3-(3-hydroxyphenyl)-N- n-propylpiperidine.

TABLE II. Antagonism of the 3-PPP-induced depression of locomotor activity in rats

Treatment	Rat locomotor activity (counts 15 min^{-1})	N
A. Glucose + physiological saline	117 ± 17	6
B. Haloperidol + physiological saline	140 ± 22	5
C. Glucose + 3-PPP	43 ± 9	5
D. Haloperidol + 3-PPP	80 ± 10***	7

Rats were given haloperidol (0.02 mg kg^{-1} i.p.) or vehicle (5.5% glucose sol.) 20 min before 3-PPP (0.5 mg kg^{-1} s.c.). 5 min later they were placed in the motility boxes and the locomotor activity during the consecutive 15 min was recorded. Shown are the means ± SEM. Statistical significances were calculated by student's t-test. *** $P < 0.025$ v. group C. (From Ref. 7.)

Fig. 3). Both the behavioural action and the effect on dopa formation are blocked by haloperidol pretreatment (Table II).

The 3-PPP-induced decrease in DA-synthesis rate is still present after γ-butyrolactone (GBL)-induced cessation of the firing in central DA neurons and can be blocked by haloperidol, thus again confirming involvement of DA receptors (Table III). The GBL-induced nerve-impulse inhibition precludes the involvement of a feedback loop. Hence, the ability of DA-receptor agonists like e.g. apomorphine and 3-PPP to antagonize the GBL-induced increase in DA-synthesis is probably due to stimulation of the DA-autoreceptors located in the terminal areas of the DA-neurons. However, since recordings of single dopaminergic neurons in the substantia nigra demonstrate cessation of firing after treatment of 3-PPP, the DA autoreceptors located on dopaminergic cell bodies are probably also stimulated by this agent.

In intact rats 3-PPP does not cause any catalepsy. This is in contrast to the action of classical neuroleptics and suggests that 3-PPP has but slight influence on extrapyramidal motor functions. The biochemical counterpart of this behavioural profile, i.e. inhibition of exploratory activity and absence of catalepsy, is an observed trend to regional selectivity, i.e. a markedly stronger inhibition of dopa formation and depression of DOPAC levels in the limbic forebrain than in the striatum.

Structure–activity relationships

A large number of analogues of 3-PPP have been studied by our group and some representative compounds are presented in Table IV. (For an extensive structure–activity relationship (SAR)-presentation, see Ref. 8.)

Variation of the position of the hydroxyl group on the aromatic ring, giving the 2-hydroxy and 4-hydroxy isomers **I** and **III**, resulted in inactive compounds. A number of derivatives with substituents other than hydroxyl in the 3-position of the aromatic ring were also studied. All these com-

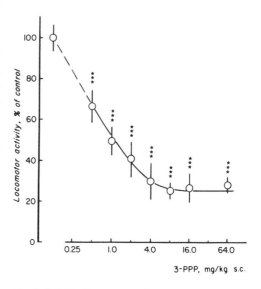

Fig. 2. 3-PPP: Suppression of rat locomotor activity. Rats were given 3-PPP (0.5–64 mg kg^{-1} s.c.). 5 min later they were placed in the motility boxes and the locomotor activity during the initial 30 min were recorded. Shown are the means ± SEM (N=3–7) % of controls. Statistical significance was reached at all dose levels (Student's t-test). (Ref. 7.)

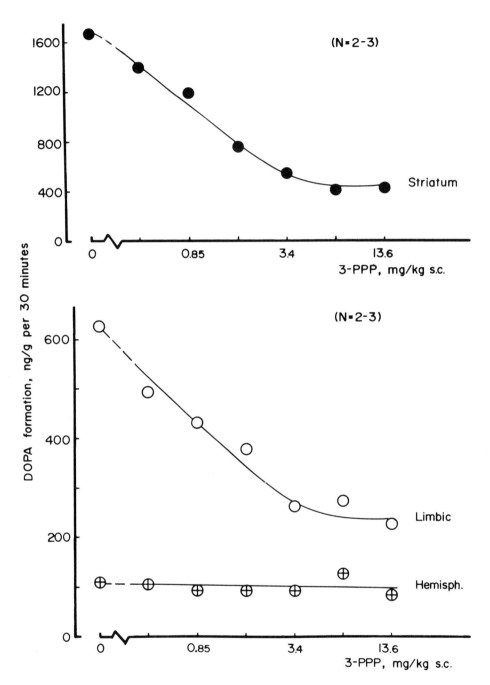

Fig. 3. 3-PPP: Effects on dopamine-synthesis rate. Rats pretreated with reserpine (5 mg kg^{-1} i.p., 18 h) were given 3-PPP (several dose levels, s.c.) 75 min prior to death, followed 45 min later by NSD 1015 (m-hydroxybenzyl-hydrazine hydrochloride, 100 mg kg^{-1} i.p., 30 min prior to death) and the brain dopa levels were determined. Shown are the medians (Ref. 7).

Explanation: *NSD 1015 is an inhibitor of the aromatic L-amino acid decarboxylase. In those areas where dopamine is the predominating catecholamine, i.e. striatum and limbic forebrain, dopa formation is markedly reduced. In the remaining part of the hemispheres (=hemisph.), where noradrenaline predominates, the dopa level is unaffected.*

TABLE III. Antagonism of 3-PPP-induced reversal of the GBL-elicited increase in DA-synthesis rate

Treatment	Dopa ng g^{-1}		N
	Limbic system	Striatum	
A. Control	307 ± 13	860 ± 40	18
B. GBL	506 ± 24	2366 ± 103	18
C. 3-PPP + GBL	191 ± 16***	1063 ± 74***	5
D. Haloperidol + 3-PPP + GBL	387 ± 32	2193 ± 53	3

Rats were given 3-PPP (32 mg kg^{-1}, s.c.) 40 min, and GBL (750 mg kg^{-1}, i.p.) 35 min before death. Haloperidol (1 mg kg^{-1}, i.p.) was given 60 min before death. All animals were given NSD 1015 (100 mg kg^{-1}, i.p.) 30 min before death, and the means ± SEM are shown. Statistical significances were calculated by student's t-test.
*** $P < 0.001$ v. GBL controls (B) as well as haloperidol-pretreated rats (D).

pounds were inactive. Taken together, the results indicate that monosubstitution with a 3-hydroxy group is an essential requirement in the 3-phenylpiperidine series to obtain a selective DA-autoreceptor stimulating compound.

The structurally related compounds 3-PPP (**II**) and 3 - hydroxy - N,N - di - n - propylphenethylamine (**XIV**) had the same order of potency in the biochemical test, both being somewhat more active than their 3,4-dihydroxy analogues (Table IV and Ref. 6). These data suggest that the DA-autoreceptors are similarly affected by the phenethylamine and 3-phenylpiperidine derivatives.

TABLE IV. Screening data for 3-PPP and some of its congeners

Compound No.	R$_1$	R$_2$	ED$_{50}$ μmol kg^{-1}	
			Limbic	Striatum
I	2-OH	n-Pr	1^a	1^a
II (3-PPP)	3-OH	n-Pr	3.6	3.6
III	4-OH	n-Pr	1	1
IV	3-OMe	n-Pr	1	1
V	3-NH$_2$	n-Pr	1	1
VI	3-CH$_2$OH	n-Pr	1	1
VII	3,4-(OH)$_2$	n-Pr	10	13^b
VIII	3-OH	H	25	25
IX	3-OH	Me	2.8	2.5
X	3-OH	Et	5.7	6.3
XI	3-OH	i-Pr	1.0	0.9
XII	3-OH	n-Bu	1.1	0.9
XIII	3-OH	-CH$_2$CH$_2$Ph	0.2	0.3^c
XIV			0.9	0.8^b

^{a} Inactive at doses > 45 μmol kg^{-1}.
^{b} Post-synaptic active.
^{c} The rats died in convulsions at a s.c. dose of 20 μmol kg^{-1}. This agent appears to stimulate post-synaptic DA receptors, as indicated by increased motility of reserpine-treated rats.

The post-synaptic DA receptors, however, seem to have different structural requirements, since they were activated by the phenethylamine **XIV** but not by 3-PPP. This may indicate that part of the piperidine ring of 3-PPP not included in the phenethylamine derivatives, is somehow responsible for the selectivity of 3-PPP. Interestingly, introduction of an additional hydroxyl group in the 4-position of the phenyl moiety seems to outweigh the effect of the piperidine ring as shown by compound **VII** which readily antagonized the reserpine-induced immobility in rats. In the present series of compounds, the structure–activity relation for the *N*-substituent seems to be complex (see compounds **VIII–XIII**). The *N-iso*-propyl-(**XI**), *N-n*-butyl-(**XII**), and *N*-phenethyl **XIII** substituted derivatives are all more potent than 3-PPP. In contrast to this, it has been shown that at least one of the *N*-substituents for the 2-amino-5-hydroxytetralin series must be smaller than *n*-butyl and should preferably be an *n*-propyl for high DA-autoreceptor stimulating activity[9]. However, the other *N*-substituent could be varied considerably without significant loss in activity. Consequently, the *N*-substituent in the 2-aminotetralin series on which less structural requirements are imposed may correspond to the *N*-substituent of the 3-phenylpiperidines.

In conclusion, our SAR-data indicate that 3-PPP and some of its analogues exhibit the profile of selective DA-autoreceptor agonists. The more precise characterization of the action of 3-PPP at the molecular level must await further studies. To this end, the resolution of the racemic mixture of 3-PPP may prove essential.

It is interesting to note that Gooddale *et al.*[10] recently reported 6,7-dihydroxy-2-(dimethylamino)tetralin (TL 99) to be a selective agonist for DA-autoreceptors, although this compound and 3-PPP have no obvious structural features in common separating them from their less selective analogues.

3-PPP seems to be the first reported apparently selective dopaminergic autoreceptor agonist. Needless to say, it will be of considerable interest to explore this new principle for studying the functions of dopamine further, especially with respect to mental functions in man. Hopefully, it will open up possibilities to achieve an antipsychotic action without extrapyramidal side effects. The serious problem of irreversible tardive dyskinesia induced by the classical neuroleptics may thus be avoided.

Reading list

1 Usdin, E. and Burmey, W. E. (eds) (1975) *Pre- and Post-synaptic Receptors*, Dekker, New York
2 Hanson, G., Alphs, L., Pradhan, S. and Lovenberg, W. (1981) *Neuropharmacology* 20, 541–548
3 Tamminga, C. A., Schaffer, M. H., Smith, R. C. and Davis, J. M. (1978) *Science* 200, 567–568
4 Smith, R. C., Tamminga, C. and Davis, J. M. (1977) *J. Neural Transm.* 40, 171–176
5 Seeman, P. (1980) *Pharmacol. Rev.* 32, 229–313
6 Wikström, H., Lindberg, P., Martinson, P., Hjorth, S., Carlsson, A., Hacksell, U., Svensson, U. and Nilsson, J. L. G. (1978) *J. Med. Chem.* 21, 864–867
7 Hjorth, S., Carlsson, A., Wikström, H., Lindberg, P., Sanchez, D., Hacksell, U., Arvidsson, L.-E., Svensson, U. and Nilsson, J. L. G. (1981) *Life Sci.* 28, 1225–1232
8 Hacksell, U., Arvidsson, L.-E., Svensson, U., Nilsson, J. L. G., Sanchez, D., Wikström, H., Lindberg, P., Hjorth, S. and Carlsson, A. *J. Med. Chem.* (in press)
9 Hacksell, U., Svensson, U., Nilsson, J. L. G., Hjorth, S., Carlsson, A., Wikström, H., Lindberg, P. and Sanchez, D. (1979) *J. Med. Chem.* 22, 1469–1475
10 Gooddale, D. B., Rusterholz, D. B., Long, J. P., Flynn, J. R., Walsh, B., Cannon, J. G. and Lee, T. (1980) *Science* 210, 1141–1143

Benzodiazepine receptors: are there endogenous ligands in the brain?

H. Möhler

Pharmaceutical Research Department, F. Hoffmann-La Roche & Co., Ltd., CH-4002 Basle, Switzerland.

In analogy to the identification of morphine receptors in the brain and the subsequent isolation of opioid peptides, the discovery of benzodiazepine receptors[1,2] has prompted a search for endogenous brain constituents, which may interact with benzodiazepine receptors and thus possibly clarify their physiological role. It was hoped that such compounds would provide new molecular terms for the description of brain function and of those diseases which are ameliorated by benzodiazepine treatment like insomnia, anxiety states, muscle spasms or convulsions. This article examines the concept of endogenous ligands and reviews the attempts to isolate them.

Benzodiazepine receptors in the CNS

The main central effects of benzodiazepines such as their anxiolytic, hypnotic, anticonvulsant and muscle relaxant effects, result primarily from an enhancement of GABAergic synaptic transmission in the CNS[5]. The effects are initiated by the interaction of benzodiazepines with specific neuronal membrane proteins, the benzodiazepine receptors. They are localized in synapses[3] which, at least in part, could be identified immunocytochemically as GABAergic[4]. Although a presynaptic localization of these receptors on GABA neurons cannot be excluded, there is evidence that they are part of the postsynaptic GABA-receptor unit which is operative in the generation of the synaptic potential. The GABA receptor unit can be pictured as a supramolecular complex containing functionally related macromolecules such as the the GABA receptor, its associated chloride (Cl)-ionophore, the benzodiazepine receptor and other proteins. The GABA-dependent activation of the Cl-ionophore may be modulated allosterically: activation of the benzodiazepine receptor leads to an enhancement of the GABA response. It should be kept in mind that benzodiazepine receptors might, in addition, occur in non-GABA-ergic synapses.

Possible physiological roles of benzodiazepine receptors

Besides their role as drug receptors, the benzodiazepine receptors may serve as targets for a physiological ligand. Two types of endogenous ligands may be found. (1) The benzodiazepine binding site may be the target for a freely diffusable compound, in particular a synaptically released neurotransmitter (neuromodulator). (2) The benzodiazepine binding site may be part of a protein interface in the GABA receptor unit, implicating the membrane protein adjacent to the benzodiazepine binding site as its endogenous ligand.

Benzodiazepine receptors as neurotransmitter (neuromodulator) receptors

If a benzodiazepine receptor is pictured as a neurotransmitter receptor, the endogenous ligand should meet criteria such as synthesis in specific neurons, release upon depolarization, interaction with the receptor and inactivation. In the case of those benzodiazepine receptors which are localized in GABAergic synapses the endogenous ligand might be a co-transmitter of GABA. In correspondence to benzodiazepines, such a compound may not elicit a synaptic response by itself but rather modulate the GABAergic synaptic transmission.

In pharmacological tests the endogenous ligand should mimic the effects of benzodiazepines such as their anticonflict, anticonvulsant, muscle relaxant and hypnotic action, provided the ligand shows the same receptor specificity as a benzodiazepine.

Recently, specific benzodiazepine antagonists were synthesized. They act at the receptor level and selectively block all the major central actions of benzodiazepines. These compounds are inactive *per se* in all neuropharmacological tests of benzodiazepines and show no overt behavioural effects in animals or man[6]. Thus, the endogenous ligand is unlikely to be a benzodiazepine antagonist.

Benzodiazepine receptors as part of a protein interface

Conceivably, the benzodiazepine binding site is not a target for an endogenous ligand of the neurotransmitter (neuromodulator)-type but rather part of a protein interface in the GABA receptor unit. A classical example of the interaction of a small effector-molecule with a protein

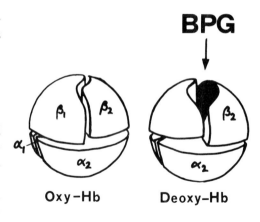

Fig. 1. Hemoglobin as a model for the interaction of a small effector molecule with a protein interface: 2,3-bisphosphoglycerate (BPG) is bound in the cleft between the two β-subunits of deoxyhemoglobin and thereby modifies the oxygen transport characteristics of hemoglobin. In analogy, benzodiazepines may be bound in a protein interface of the GABA receptor unit; the endogenous ligand may be a membrane protein interacting with the benzodiazepine binding site.

interface is provided by hemoglobin (Fig. 1). When oxyhemoglobin is deoxygenated, a rearrangement of the hemoglobin subunits occurs which includes the opening of a gap between the two β-subunits. This cleft in the deoxyhemoglobin is tailormade to fit the molecule 2,3-bisphosphoglycerate (BPG), a physiological constituent of erythrocytes. BPG is bound to the protein surface lining the cleft, stabilizes the deoxyhemoglobin conformation and thereby reduces the affinity of hemoglobin for oxygen. (Upon oxygenation of deoxyhemoglobin, BPG is extruded because the cleft becomes too small, its binding site is masked in the interface of the β-subunits of oxyhemoglobin).

Similarly, the benzodiazepine binding site may be part of a protein interface in the GABA receptor unit. The protein which contacts the benzodiazepine receptor in this interface might function as an endogenous ligand to the benzodiazepine binding site. In the presence of benzodiazepines the dynamics of the protein–protein interaction would be altered resulting in an enhancement of the GABA response.

Depending on the conformational state of the GABA receptor unit, benzodiazepine binding sites may be exposed or masked. This would be in line with the finding that the number of accessible benzodiazepine binding sites can be rapidly altered by various treatments e.g. by either chemically or electrically induced seizures[7]. The malfunction of protein interactions in GABA receptor units may be the basis of at least some diseases which are ameliorated by benzodiazepine treatment.

Putative endogenous ligands

Nearly all research groups involved used the same approach in the search for endogenous ligands. Extracts of brain tissue were fractionated in various ways and tested for their ability to displace [³H]diazepam from the benzodiazepine receptor in brain membrane fragments. The following compounds have so far been proposed as putative endogenous ligands (Fig. 2): inosine, hypoxanthine, nicotinamide, ethyl-β-carboline-3-carboxylate and various proteins including GABA-modulin. Thromboxane A₂ was also suggested as a candidate. The characteristics of these compounds are described in the following section.

Purines and purine nucleosides

Inosine and hypoxanthine (Fig. 2), the first candidates of this group of compounds, can be released from brain slices by K+ depolarization. Their affinity to the benzodiazepine receptor is however rather poor[8,9,10]. About 1 mM concentration is needed for half maximal inhibition of [³H]diazepam binding *in vitro*, indicating

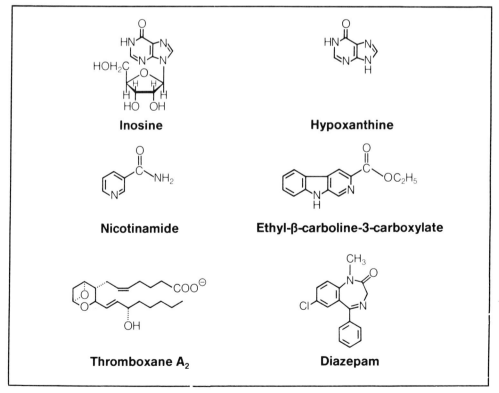

Fig. 2. Putative endogenous benzodiazepine receptor ligands with known chemical structure. Diazepam is shown for comparison.

that the affinity of either compound to the receptor is about 200,000 times less than that of diazepam. The pharmacological evaluation of the two purine compounds is hampered by their poor penetration into the brain after systemic application. After 1000 mg kg^{-1} i.p., hypoxanthine showed a slight protective effect against seizures induced by 3-mercaptopropionic acid in mice[10]. After intraventricular administration, inosine increased the latency of seizures induced by pentylenetetrazole while pyrimidines or other purines which were ineffective in inhibiting [^{3}H]diazepam binding *in vitro* were without effect on seizure latency[8]. Electrophysiologically, conflicting results have been found. In primary cultures of mouse spinal cord, inosine and flurazepam elicited a rapid excitatory response showing cross-desensitization, which indicates that both compounds affect the same conductance mechanism. An additional slow inhibitory response of inosine was blocked by flurazepam[11]. *In vivo*, in recordings of cat spinal cord activities, inosine and hypoxanthine did not exert benzodiazepine-like effects, when applied *in situ* by pressure ejection from a cannula[10]; the purine concentrations used were the same as those for nicotinamide, which elicited benzodiazepine-like effects despite its somewhat lower affinity to the benzodiazepine receptor (see below).

Among the structurally related purine derivatives guanosine has the same affinity to the benzodiazepine receptor as inosine and hypoxanthine while adenosine has a five times lower affinity[9]. The depressant action of adenosine on spontaneous firing of rat cerebral cortical neurons could be potentiated by diazepam and the depressant action of flurazepam could be antagonized by theophylline, an adenosine antagonist. These findings lead to the interesting notion that benzodiazepine receptors may, at least in part, correspond to uptake sites for adenosine and possibly other purine nucleosides[12].

At present, however, the evidence for a role of purines and purine nucleosides as endogenous benzodiazepine receptor ligands is not compelling. In particular, it is not known if the sites of release of these compounds correspond to the localization of benzodiazepine receptors in the brain. Furthermore, apart from anticonvulsant effects, the presumptive benzodiazepine-like neuropharmacological profile of these compounds remains to be established.

Nicotinamide

Nicotinamide (Fig. 2) is formed in the brain by enzymatic hydrolysis of nicotinamide-adenine-dinucleotide (NAD). Furthermore ADP-ribosylation processes may lead to the formation of nicotinamide from NAD. The affinity of nicotinamide to the benzodiazepine receptor *in vitro* is rather poor with half maximal inhibition of [^{3}H]diazepam binding *in vitro* occurring at 4 mM. However, as in the case of purine derivatives, the low affinity does not preclude a biological action, since high local concentrations of the compounds may occur and activation of only a small percentage of receptors may be sufficient. Nicotinamide showed the main neuropharmacological central effects characteristic of a benzodiazepine[10]. Nicotinamide, (1) suppressed seizures induced by 3-mercaptopropionic acid in mice, (2) restored punishment-suppressed behaviour in rats, an action characteristic of anti-anxiety agents, (3) inhibited aggressive rage reactions in cats elicited by hypothalamic electrical stimulation, (4) showed muscle relaxant action in several species, (5) resulted in hypnotic action in mice and man by increasing both total sleep time and REM sleep, and (6) mimicked the action of diazepam on GABA turnover in various brain areas of stressed animals[10,13]. In these experiments 300–500 mg kg^{-1} i.p.

were usually administered due to the poor penetration of nicotinamide into the brain. In electrophysiological experiments in cat spinal cord *in vivo*, nicotinamide was applied *in situ* through a cannula by pressure ejection. It elicited effects which were very similar in size and latency to those found with a very potent benzodiazepine applied in the same way and concentration. The effects were reversed by (+)bicuculline[10]. These results document the benzodiazepine-like action of nicotinamide. Most conspicuously, the potency of nicotinamide after *in situ* application was equivalent to that of a highly potent benzodiazepine[10]. These findings are in line with a possible role of nicotinamide as endogenous benzodiazepine receptor ligand. At present, however, it is not known if nicotinamide is released from brain cells, in particular from cells near benzodiazepine receptors.

Thromboxane A₂

From experiments with a rat vascular preparation in which the vasoconstrictor effect of thromboxane A₂ was antagonized by diazepam and chlordiazepoxide, it was proposed that thromboxane A₂ may be an endogenous ligand to the benzodiazepine receptor in the brain[14]. So far, however, there is no experimental evidence that thromboxane A₂ interacts with the central type of benzodiazepine receptor and elicits central benzodiazepine-like actions. The extreme instability of thromboxane A₂ poses problems not only in experiments but also for a possible neurotransmitter role (storage) of the compound. Its half-life is $t_{1/2} = 30$ sec at 37°C, pH 7.4.

Ethyl-β-carboline-3-carboxylate (γ-substance)

This compound is of pharmacological interest since it binds to the benzodiazepine receptor with high affinity; half-maximal inhibition of [³H]flunitrazepam binding *in vitro* occurs at a concentration of 7 nM[15]. Neuropharmacologically the substance lowers the seizure threshold to pentylenetetrazol and reverses at least some benzodiazepine actions. However, the compound is possibly not a brain constituent, but rather a product formed during tissue extraction. The procedure included treatment of brain (or urine) fractions with 99.9% ethanol/3% concentrated HC1 for 20 h at 80°C[15]. It is known that under hydrolysing conditions, β-carbolines are formed from tryptophan containing proteins. In the presence of ethanol an ethylester will be found. So far, the compound could not be isolated with other procedures. It can, however, not be excluded that some other β-carboline derivatives may play a physiological role by interacting with benzodiazepine receptors.

Peptides and proteins

Various brain fractions contained inhibitory activity of [³H]diazepam binding which was susceptible to proteolysis[16,17,18]. These presumptive peptides and proteins span a wide range of mol. wts (1500 to 40,000–70,000). At least some of the high molecular weight compounds may be part of the GABA receptor unit. This seems to be the case for GABA-modulin[16], a protein isolated from synaptic membrane fractions by Triton treatment; it inhibits competitively not only [³H]diazepam binding but also the high affinity GABA receptor binding. Thus, GABA-modulin appears to be a building block of the GABA receptor unit interacting with the benzodiazepine binding site either indirectly through an allosteric mechanism or directly at the recognition site. In the latter case GABA-modulin may be considered as an endogenous ligand to the benzodiazepine receptor.

Other presumptive polypeptides may be benzodiazepine receptor ligands or their precursors. However, at present, their characterization and their localization in the brain is not sufficient to allow an assessment of a possible physiological role in connection with benzodiazepine receptors.

Other hitherto less well characterized inhibitors of [^{3}H]diazepam binding seem to be present in the brain[19,20].

Summary

The search goes on. There is as yet no compelling evidence for the existence of an endogenous benzodiazepine receptor ligand in the brain. At present, nicotinamide appears to be a very promising candidate in view of its benzodiazepine-like neuropharmacological profile. Purine derivatives also have to be considered as putative endogenous ligands. Alternatively, the endogenous ligand may not be a neurotransmitter (neuromodulator)-type compound but a membrane protein, in particular, a constituent of GABA receptor units. In the future, the search will become more selective: the recently discovered benzodiazepine antagonists[6] will help to specify whether a response of a putative endogenous ligand is mediated via the benzodiazepine receptor or not. However, it should be kept in mind that drug receptors are not necessarily target sites for a physiological ligand.

Reading list

1 Möhler, H. and Okada, T. (1977) *Science* 198, 849–851
2 Squires, R. F. and Braestrup, C. (1977) *Nature (London)* 266, 732–734
3 Möhler, H., Battersby, M. K. and Richards, J. G. (1980) *Proc. Natl Acad. Sci. U.S.A.* 77, 1666–1670
4 Möhler, H., Richards, J. G. and Wu, Y. J. (1981) *Proc. Natl Acad. Sci. U.S.A.* 78, 1935–1938
5 Haefely, W., Polc, P., Schaffner, R., Keller, H., Pieri, L. and Möhler, H. (1978) in *GABA-Neurotransmitters* (Krogsgaard-Larson, P., Scheel-Krüger, J. and Kofod, H., eds), pp. 357–375, Munksgaard, Copenhagen
6 Hunkeler, W., Möhler, H., Pieri, L., Polc, P., Bonetti, E. P., Cumin, R., Schaffner, R. and Haefely, W. (1981) *Nature (London)* 290, 514–516
7 Paul, S. M. and Skolnick, P. (1978) *Science* 202, 892–893
8 Skolnick, P., Syapin, P. J., Paugh, B. A., Moncada, V., Marangos, P. J. and Paul, S. M. (1979) *Proc. Natl Acad. Sci. U.S.A.* 76, 1515–1518
9 Asano, T. and Spector, S. (1979) *Proc. Natl Acad. Sci. U.S.A.* 76, 977–981
10 Möhler, H., Polc, P., Cumin, R., Pieri, L. and Kettler, R. (1979) *Nature (London)* 278, 563–565
11 McDonald, J. F., Barker, J. L., Paul, S. M. and Marangos, P. J. (1979) *Science* 205, 715–717
12 Wu, P. H., Phillis, J. W. and Bender, A. S. (1980) *Eur. J. Pharmacol.* 65, 459–460
13 Kennedy, B. and Leonard, B. E. (1980) *Biochem. Soc. Trans.* 8, 59–60
14 Ally, A. I., Manku, M. S., Horrobin, D. F., Karmali, R. A., Morgan, R. O. and Marmazyn, M. (1978) *Neurosci. Lett.* 7, 31–34
15 Braestrup, C., Nielsen, M. and Olsen, C. E. (1980) *Proc. Natl Acad. Sci. U.S.A.* 77, 2288–2292
16 Guidotti, A., Toffano, G. and Costa, E. (1978) *Nature (London)* 275, 553–555
17 Colello, G. D., Hockenbery, D. M., Bosmann, H. M., Fuchs, S. and Folkers, K. (1978) *Proc. Natl Acad. Sci. U.S.A.* 75, 6319–6323
18 Davis, L. G. and Cohen, R. K. (1980) *Biochem. Biophys. Res. Commun.* 92, 141–148
19 Karobath, M., Sperk, G. and Schönbeck, G. (1978) *Eur. J. Pharmacol.* 49, 323–326
20 Poddar, M. K., Urquhart, D. and Sinha, A. K. (1980) *Brain Res.* 193, 519–528

GABA and barbiturate receptors

Graham A. R. Johnston and Max Willow

Department of Pharmacology, University of Sydney, NSW 2006, Australia

Barbiturates potentiate GABA-mediated synaptic transmission in many areas of the CNS. Recent results from studies on the binding of radioactive GABA and phenobarbitone indicate that barbiturates act on a distinct class of receptors to decrease the rate of dissociation of GABA from certain receptors for this major inhibitory transmitter.

Anaesthetic and anticonvulsant barbiturates enhance synaptic transmission mediated by 4-aminobutanoic acid (GABA)[1]. GABA is an inhibitory transmitter of major significance in many areas of the CNS[2,3] and enhancement of synaptic inhibition may underlie many of the pharmacological effects of these barbiturates. While there have been numerous electrophysiological studies demonstrating that barbiturates enhance neuronal responses to exogenous GABA, until recently the mechanisms which underlie the interaction between GABA and barbiturate receptors have remained unknown. Ligand binding studies using radiolabelled GABA and related compounds have provided many interesting data on the intricacies of the interactions between GABA receptors and their related chloride ionophores, a major action of GABA *in vivo* being to increase chloride permeability in post-synaptic membranes[2]. There have been many binding studies on the interactions between GABA and the benzodiazepines[2], a class of drugs which are also known to enhance GABA-mediated synaptic transmission at certain sites and which share a number of pharmacological actions with barbiturates. Until recently, however, studies of GABA binding have failed to demonstrate any effect of barbiturates. It is now apparent that the method of membrane preparation is vital for the demonstration of enhancement of GABA binding by barbiturates.

Barbiturate enhancement of GABA binding

GABA receptors on brain membranes appear to be rather robust structures and certain protocols involving freeze–thaw regimes or extraction with non-ionic detergents, such as Triton X-100, are used to maximize specific GABA binding in many experiments. It is now known that these protocols remove endogenous inhibitors of GABA binding (GABARINS) from the membranes to reveal latent binding sites[3]. These protocols appear to alter the links between GABA and barbiturate recognition sites and it is therefore necessary to use less disrupted membrane preparations in order to observe these barbiturate effects[4].

We have used a relatively crude synaptic membrane preparation from rat brain incorporating the following features: (i) gentle homogenization of brain tissue in a glass-Teflon homogenizer with a loose fitting pestle in isotonic sucrose and (ii) extended washing (8–10 times) of the P2 crude mitochondrial pellet by very careful resuspension in hypo-osmotic TRIS-citrate buffer followed by centrifugation. The binding of tritiated GABA to this preparation was studied using a centrifugation assay at 4°C. Using a 5-min incubation period in 50 mM TRIS-citrate buffer at pH 7.1. GABA binding studied in this way exhibited biphasic kinetics with apparent Kd values of 0.02 and 2.6 μM and apparent binding densities of 0.8 and 7.5 pmol mg^{-1} protein respectively for the higher and lower affinity sites, as determined by non-linear regression analysis of Scatchard plots[5]. With these membranes, we were able to show a dose-dependent enhancement of GABA binding by pentobarbitone and a number of related barbiturates. This enhancement involved an increased affinity of GABA for the higher affinity of the two apparent GABA binding sites (change in Kd from 0.02 to 0.009 μM in the presence of 100 μM pentobarbitone). There was no significant change produced by pentobarbitone in the affinity of the lower affinity sites or in the apparent densities of either class of sites.

A number of clinically useful anaesthetic/anticonvulsant barbiturates enhanced the binding of GABA to these extensively washed crude synaptic membrane preparations, producing a maximal enhancement of approximately 40%. The concentrations required to produce half maximal enhancement of GABA binding lie well within the range of concentrations of these barbiturates found in the brains of anaesthetized laboratory animals. For example, pentobarbitone produced half maximal enhancement of GABA binding at 38 μM. The short acting anaesthetic etomidate also enhanced GABA binding but acted to increase the *density* of higher affinity GABA binding sites, indicating a difference in its mechanism of action compared to that of the barbiturates[5].

Receptors and ionophores

The enhancement of GABA binding by barbiturates appears to involve a close association with GABA-related ionophores, since the enhancement can be inhibited by the ionophore antagonist picrotoxinin. Since picrotoxinin does not influence the binding of GABA to its receptors, this indicates that barbiturates do not act directly on GABA receptors to enhance GABA binding. At high concentrations (>0.5 mM), however, barbiturates do exhibit a direct GABA-mimetic effect which is not influenced by detergent extraction of the membranes. The detergent-sensitive GABA enhancement produced at low concentrations of barbiturates seems to require the coupling between certain GABA receptors and picrotoxinin-sensitive ionophores to be maintained. This coupling might be mediated via certain of the endogenous inhibitors of GABA binding that are known to be removed on detergent extraction.

Barbiturate binding sites

We have recently characterized a barbiturate binding site in the extensively washed crude synaptic membrane preparation described above. Under the same conditions used to study GABA binding and barbiturate enhancement thereof, tritiated phenobarbitone bound to a single class of sites in these membranes with a relatively low affinity (Kd 100 μM) and high density (800 pmol mg^{-1})[6]. These phenobarbitone binding sites were abolished on detergent extraction of the membranes under conditions where GABA binding was retained and facilitated. Neither GABA nor the GABA receptor antagonist, bicuculline, influenced phenobarbitone binding.

Despite our observation that picrotoxinin antagonized the enhancement of GABA binding by barbiturates, and the demonstration that barbiturates inhibit the binding of a labelled picrotoxin derivative (dihydropicrotoxinin) to synaptosomal membranes[7], the binding of phenobarbitone was not influenced by picrotoxinin.

Thus, barbiturates can potentiate GABA binding and inhibit dihydropicrotoxinin binding, whereas barbiturate binding is not influenced by activation of these other binding sites.

Phenobarbitone could be displaced from the binding sites on these membranes by a range of substituted barbiturates. There was an excellent direct correlation between the ability to displace phenobarbitone and the ability to enhance GABA binding for those barbiturates possessing anaesthetic, anticonvulsant or depressant properties in that the concentrations for half maximal displacement and half maximal enhancement were almost identical. This indicates that both phenomena are directly linked, the interaction with barbiturate binding sites resulting in enhancement of GABA binding. Both barbiturate binding and GABA enhancement were abolished on detergent extraction indicating that detergent-sensitive components were responsible for the coupling between the two classes of sites.

There is a close correlation between the octanol-water partition coefficients for these barbiturates and their ability to enhance GABA binding and to displace phenobarbitone binding. Lipids may be important components of GABA receptor complexes with phospholipids such as phosphatidylethanolamine acting as endogenous inhibitors of GABA binding[3]. Detergent extraction is known to remove some phospholipids from synaptic membranes and it may well be that the barbiturate binding sites have phospholipid components. This may account for the apparent high density of phenobarbitone binding sites measured on the basis of protein concentration. If these membrane binding sites are in part lipid in nature then this would tend to support certain aspects of the Meyer–Overton hypothesis regarding anaesthetics and membrane lipids. At the turn of the century, Meyer and Overton proposed that anaesthesia resulted from an interaction of the drug with the lipids of cell membranes thus stabilizing the structure of neuronal membranes by packing into the lipid layer. We would propose that barbiturates interact with specific phospholipid structures to enhance the binding of GABA to certain of its receptors, perhaps via a change in membrane fluidity.

Barbiturates decrease the rate of dissociation of GABA

The apparent increase in affinity of GABA for the higher affinity binding sites in the crude synaptic membranes induced by barbiturates may be accounted for by a decrease in the rate of dissociation of GABA from these sites[8]. This would be expected to increase the life time of barbiturate-coupled GABA-receptor complexes and would be consistent with the observed increased life time of GABA-activated chloride channels measured in cultured neurones in the presence of pentobarbitone[9].

Olsen and his colleagues have described an anion-dependent barbiturate-induced enhancement of GABA binding characterized by an apparent increase in the density of GABA sites[7]. This density effect requires a five-fold higher concentration of barbiturate than the affinity effect we have described, and is not so dependent on the mode of preparation of the membranes. An increased GABA binding density would not account for the increased life time of GABA-activated chloride channels and indeed need not necessarily result in potentiation of GABA action if spare receptors exist for GABA. However, the apparent increase in density could be due to an increase in affinity for normally undetectable low affinity GABA binding sites[7].

Multiplicity of receptors

It is becoming increasingly apparent that there is a multiplicity of GABA receptors, barbiturate receptors and benzodiazepine receptors, and that these are linked in a number of ways[3]. Thus, there are likely to be at least the following broad classes of such receptors: (i) GABA receptors that are not influenced by barbiturate or benzodiazepine receptors, (ii) GABA receptors that are linked to barbiturate receptors but not to benzodiazepine receptors, (iii) GABA receptors that are linked to benzodiazepine receptors but not to barbiturate receptors, (iv) GABA receptors that are linked to both barbiturate and benzodiazepine receptors, (v) barbiturate receptors that are not linked to GABA or benzodiazepine receptors, and (vi) benzodiazepine receptors that are not linked to GABA or barbiturate receptors.

In the present context, it is pertinent to emphasize classification (v) above, in that not all actions of barbiturates are mediated by potentiation of GABA-mediated synaptic transmission. We have studied the effects of barbiturates on a calcium-ATPase activity in synaptic membranes which seems to influence calcium movements vital to transmitter release[10]. A major action of anaesthetic/anticonvulsant barbiturates may well be inhibition of the release of excitatory transmitters.

Conclusion

Barbiturates can influence the functional state of certain complexes associated with GABA receptors, leading to a decreased rate of dissociation of GABA. This may involve a class of barbiturate receptors that are in part lipid in nature and that are removed by many of the conventional membrane preparations now used to study GABA binding.

Reading list

1 Nicoll, R. A. (1980) in *Handbook of Psychopharmacology* (Iversen, L. L., Iversen, S. D. and Snyder, S. H., eds), Vol. 12, pp. 187–234, Plenum Press, New York
2 Enna, S. J. (1981) *Trends Pharmacol. Sci.* 2, 62–64
3 Johnston, G. A. R. (1981) in *The Role of Peptides and Amino Acids as Neurotransmitters* (Lombardini, J. B. and Kenny, A. D., eds), pp. 3–17, Alan Liss, New York
4 Willow, M. and Johnston, G. A. R. (1981) *J. Neurosci.* 1, 364–367
5 Willow, M. (1981) *Brain Res.* 220, 427–431
6 Willow, M., Morgan, I. G. and Johnston, G. A. R. (1981) *Neurosci. Lett.* 24, 301–306
7 Olsen, R. W. (1981) *J. Neurochem.* 37, 1–13
8 Willow, M. and Johnston, G. A. R. (1981) *Neurosci. Lett.* 23, 71–74
9 Barker, J. L. and Mathers, D. A. (1981) *Trends NeuroSci.* 4, 10–13
10 Willow, M., Bornstein, I. C. and Johnston, G. A. R. (1980) *Neurosci. Lett.* 18, 323–327

Physiological consequences of muscarinic receptor activation

H. Criss Hartzell

Department of Anatomy, Emory University School of Medicine, Atlanta, GA 30322, U.S.A.

Recent studies on muscarinic acetylcholine (ACh) receptors have shown that these receptors differ in very important and fundamental ways from the more extensively studied nicotinic ACh receptors. Muscarinic receptors are coupled to several different types of ionic channels in the plasma membrane by a process which probably involves a series of three or more steps. Some of these steps may involve enzymatic processes. In addition to being coupled to conventional drug-activated ionic channels which are not affected by membrane potential, muscarinic receptors are capable of modulating the opening and closing of channels which are gated by changes in transmembrane potential. Activation of muscarinic receptors also produces a variety of metabolic responses in post-synaptic cells that may be important in mediating long-term signalling between neurones and their targets.

Receptors for ACh can be divided into two broad categories, muscarinic and nicotinic. The distinction between these receptors was first made on empirical, pharmacological grounds: certain responses to ACh, such as the endplate potential of skeletal muscle, were mimicked by *nicotine* and blocked by curare, whereas other responses, such as the inhibitory effect of ACh on the heart beat, were mimicked by *muscarine* and blocked by atropine. Recently, however, it has become clear that muscarinic and nicotinic receptors differ in more interesting ways than just their affinity for agonists and antagonists. Indeed, the molecular mechanisms coupling these receptors to their physiological responses are fundamentally different. Nicotinic ACh receptors (nAChR) are directly and permanently coupled to the ionic channels they control, but muscarinic ACh receptors (mAChR) are indirectly or transiently coupled to their channels. Furthermore, mAChR produce a variety of biochemical responses in the cell that are not produced by nicotinic actions of ACh.

Coupling of receptors to channels

The idea that nAChR are permanently coupled to their channels comes from the observation that all nicotinic receptors which have been examined produce the same kind of post-synaptic response, a rather non-selective increase in permeability to small cations resulting in a depolarizing excitatory post-synaptic potential (e.p.s.p.). It is very likely that the ionic channel and the nicotinic ACh binding site are parts of the same macromolecular complex[1] because the ionic permeability of artificial membrane bilayers containing purified nAChR can be regulated by ACh[2].

It is postulated that binding of ACh to the receptor produces a conformational change in the molecule and that this change is the opening of the ionic channel.

Muscarinic receptors, in contrast, mediate a variety of different conductance changes in different cells. This suggests that the muscarinic ACh binding sites are located on molecules different from the ionic channels. mAChR are often coupled to several types of channels in the same cell. For example, in cardiac muscle cells mAChR are coupled to both K^+ and Ca^{2+} channels. When ACh is applied to cardiac muscle, there are two effects[3]: (a) an increase in background K conductance (g_K), resulting in membrane hyperpolarization and slowing of the heartbeat and (b) a decrease in the Ca^{2+} influx which occurs during the action potential, resulting in decreased contractile force. Another interesting example has been studied in amphibian sympathetic neurones where ACh produces two responses having different time courses and opposite ionic mechanisms[4]. In these cells, muscarinic agonists evoke a slow inhibitory postsynaptic potential (i.p.s.p.) followed by a slower e.p.s.p. The slow i.p.s.p. is produced by opening of K^+ channels[5,6] and the slow e.p.s.p. is due to the closing of a different kind of K^+ channel called the M-channel[7]. The M-channel has characteristics which distinguish it from other known K^+ channels in this neurone. M-channels are open at depolarized membrane potentials but are closed at membrane potentials negative to -60 mV. ACh closes the M-channels which have been opened by membrane depolarization. Thus, at depolarized potentials, ACh depolarizes the cell further by turning off the M-current which is drawing the membrane potential toward E_K.

These examples illustrate several important features of muscarinic responses which have recently been recognized. Some muscarinic responses (such as the increase in g_K in heart and the slow i.p.s.p. in the neurone) occur by classical ionic mechanisms: ACh opens ionic channels which are normally closed and have relatively little voltage sensitivity. Other muscarinic responses (such as the effect on Ca^{2+} influx in heart and on M-channels in the neurone), however, involve channels which are also gated by membrane voltage. Classically, ionic channels have been divided into ones which are gated by transmembrane potential ('Hodgkin–Huxley' type channels, for example) and channels which are gated by neurotransmitters (e.g. nicotinic channels). The muscarinic regulation of channels which are also voltage-sensitive provides a powerful mechanism whereby ACh can modulate electrical excitability and synaptic function without necessarily producing a change in resting membrane potential.

What is the mechanism by which mAChR are coupled to different classes of channels? One possibility is that there are subclasses of mAChR, each of which is coupled permanently to a different ionic channel. Although Birdsall et al.[8] have shown that mAChR can be subdivided into several classes on the basis of their affinity for the muscarinic agonist [^{3}H]oxotremorine-M, difficulties are encountered in determining which of these classes are related to physiological responses. Giles and Noble[3] have demonstrated that the concentration of ACh required to decrease Ca^{2+} influx in heart cells is smaller than the concentration required to affect g_K. An interpretation of this finding is that different subclasses of mAChR having different affinities for ACh mediate these two different conductance changes.

Coupling mechanisms

There are several reasons, however, to think that the coupling mechanisms for mAChR and nAChR are fundamentally different[9]. (i) Muscarinic responses last much longer than nicotinic responses. For example, a 1-ms duration ACh pulse produces a response in skeletal muscle that lasts 10 ms, but the same pulse of ACh evokes a response in cardiac muscle that is about $1000\times$ slower[9]. This longer duration is not simply due to a longer mean open time of the individual ionic channels. Recent measurements of ACh induced noise in the rabbit sino-atrial node in Trautwein's laboratory[10], and single channel measurements of ACh channels in embryonic chick atrium in my own laboratory (unpublished) have shown that channel open time is short (~ 100 ms) relative to the time course of the response to ACh (seconds). Thus, muscarinic channels must be repeatedly activated during the decay of the response[9]. This is in contrast to nicotinic channels which are opened only once in response to a brief pulse of ACh. The mechanism of repeated channel activation is not known but might involve slow dissociation of ACh from receptors, repeated ACh binding, or the slow decline of second messenger concentration which is responsible for channel activation. (ii) The onset of the response to muscarinic agents is too slow to be explained by a simple two-step model for channel activation[9,11,12]. For example, activation of nicotinic channels can be described by the scheme:

$$nACh + R \underset{\text{fast}}{\xrightleftharpoons{\text{binding}}} ACh_n R$$

$$ACh_n R \underset{\text{rate-limiting}}{\xrightleftharpoons{\text{isomerization}}} (ACh_n R)^*$$

where n molecules of ACh bind to a receptor very quickly and the channel then changes conformation (isomerization) and opens. Channel opening is the rate-limiting step. In this scheme, brief pulses of ACh are expected to produce a rapid, exponential change in membrane conductance, which is observed at the motor endplate. Muscarinic responses, however, usually begin with a 50–200 ms lag period after application of ACh and have a sigmoid rising phase[9,12,13]. These kinetics suggest that there are multiple steps between binding and isomerization. Several different multi-step models have been proposed.

The subunit hypothesis[11] supposes that ACh molecules must be bound to several receptors before a channel will open. The slow onset of the muscarinic response is explained by assuming that several ACh-receptor complexes must interact with one another for a channel to open. Interaction between subunits depends upon their diffusion and collision with one another in the membrane.

The second messenger model hypothesizes that the ACh binding site is indirectly coupled to the ionic channel by an intracellular, diffusible chemical which accumulates in response to transmitter binding and is somehow responsible for channel opening. For example, it has been proposed that the slow e.p.s.p. in sympathetic neurones is mediated by cyclic GMP[14]. Binding of ACh to mAChR activates guanylate cyclase and elevates intracellular cyclic GMP. By analogy with the cyclic AMP system, it is hypothesized that cyclic GMP activates a cyclic GMP-dependent protein kinase which phosphorylates ionic channels. Phosphorylation and dephosphorylation of the channel is presumed to convert the channel from closed to open conformation. Similarly, it has been suggested that the response of the heart to ACh is mediated by the cyclic GMP system[15].

Although this hypothesis is attractive because it explains how mAChRs may be coupled to different kinds of channels and because it seems to explain the slowness of the muscarinic response, evidence for the involvement of cyclic GMP is not strong. In sympathetic neurones, dibutyryl cyclic GMP produces different conductance changes than does ACh[16]. In heart muscle, it appears that some of the effects of ACh may be mediated by cyclic GMP while others are not. For example, 8-bromo cyclic GMP is capable of mimicking the effects of ACh on Ca^{2+} influx but is not

Metabolic effects

The action of ACh on cyclic GMP levels is only one example of the metabolic effects mediated by mAChR. Activation of mAChR may also lead to decreases in cyclic AMP levels and to increases in phosphatidyl inositol turnover. ACh can also regulate a variety of metabolic processes in the cell by altering the enzymatic phosphorylation of various proteins. For example, by decreasing cyclic AMP levels, ACh produces a decrease in cyclic AMP-dependent protein kinase activity and a decrease in phosphorylation of glycogen phosphorylase in heart cells[18]. This results in a decrease in glycogenolysis. In smooth muscle, the muscarinic action of ACh may stimulate the cyclic GMP-dependent phosphorylation of membrane proteins[14]. Recently, we have been studying the phosphorylation and dephosphorylation of a myofibrillar protein[19], termed C-protein, which is found in the A band of the myofibril. C-protein becomes phosphorylated in response to β-adrenergic agonists[19,20] and dephosphorylated in response to muscarinic agonists[19]. The dephosphorylation produced by ACh does not seem to involve either cyclic GMP or cyclic AMP. The role of C-protein phosphorylation and dephosphorylation in regulation of the heartbeat is unknown, but the location of C-protein in the region of overlap between actin and myosin filaments is intriguing.

The finding that mAChR can regulate biochemical processes in the cell by altering the phosphorylation of proteins is very important in understanding how these receptors work. From studies on muscarinic and other types of receptors it is becoming increasingly more clear that signalling in the nervous system involves much more than changes in membrane conductance, but also involves slower changes in enzymatic processes which may be important in modulating the long-term activity of neuronal circuits.

Reading list

1 Raftery, M. A., Hunkapiller, M. W., Strader, C. D. and Hood, L. E. (1980) *Science* 208, 1454–1456
2 Nelso, N., Anholt, R., Lindstrom, J. and Montal, M. (1980) *Proc. Natl Acad. Sci. U.S.A.* 77, 3057–3061
3 Giles, W. and Noble, S. J. (1976) *J. Physiol. (London)* 261, 103–123
4 Kuba, K. and Koketsu, K. (1978) *Prog. Neurobiol.* 11, 77–169
5 Horn, J. and Dodd, J. (1981) *Nature (London)* 292, 625–627
6 Weight, F. F., Schulman, J. A., Smith, D. A. and Busin, N. A. (1979) *Fed. Proc. Fed. Am. Soc. Exp. Biol.* 38, 2084–2094
7 Brown, D. A. and Adams, P. R. (1980) *Nature (London)* 283, 673–675
8 Birdsall, N. J. M., Burgen, A. S. V. and Hulme, E. C. (1978) *Mol. Pharmacol.* 14, 723–736
9 Hartzell, H. C. (1981) *Nature (London)* 291, 539–544
10 Osterrieder, W., Noma, A. and Trautwein, W. (1980) *Pflugers Arch. Ges Physiol.* 386, 101–109
11 Kehoe, J. S. and Marty, A. A. (1980) *Rev. Biophys. Bioengng* 9, 437–465
12 Hartzell, H. C., Kuffler, S. W., Stickgold, R. and Yoshikami, D. (1977) *J. Physiol. (London)* 271, 817–846
13 Purves, R. D. (1976) *Nature (London)* 261, 149–151
14 Greengard, P. (1976) *Nature (London)* 260, 101–108
15 Linden, J. and Brooker, G. (1979) *Biochem. Pharmacol.* 28, 3351–3360
16 Dun, N. J., Kaibara, K. and Karczmar, A. G. (1978) *Brain Res.* 150, 658–661
17 Nawrath, H. (1977) *Nature (London)* 267, 72–74
18 Gardner, R. M. and Allen, D. O. (1977) *J. Pharmacol. Exp. Ther.* 202, 346–353
19 Hartzell, H. C. and Titus, L. T. *J. Biol. Chem.* (in press)
20 Jeacocke, S. A. and England, P. J. (1980) *FEBS Lett.* 122, 129–132

Biochemical studies on muscarinic receptors

Mordechai Sokolovsky and Tamas Bartfai

Department of Biochemistry, George S. Wise Faculty of Life Sciences, Tel-Aviv University, Tel Aviv, 69978 Israel, and Department of Biochemistry, Arrhenius Laboratory, University of Stockholm, S-106 91 Stockholm, Sweden.

The slow actions of acetylcholine (those with a latency of 100 ms and a duration of 300–500 ms) are mediated by muscarinic receptors located on neurons in the central nervous system (CNS) and peripheral nervous system, on muscle cells in the gut and heart and on secretory cells in the pancreas and parotid[1]. *The pharmacological characterization of muscarinic receptors is based on Dale's definition from 1914 stating that these receptors are activated by acetylcholine and muscarine and blocked by atropine. Biochemical characterization of the muscarinic receptors by binding studies using radiolabeled ligands, correlation of receptor occupancy and ion fluxes, phosphatidyl inositol turnover and stimulation of cGMP synthesis has been reported. While solubilization of this endomembrane protein has been repeatedly achieved, although in poor yield, no reconstituted muscarinic receptor system that retains functional activity has yet been reported. This review summarizes data accumulated from studies on membrane-bound receptors in intact animals, whole cells or membrane preparations.*

Ligand binding studies

Antagonist binding

^{3}H-labeled reversible antagonists with high specific activity (5–90 Ci/mmol), e.g. [^{3}H]atropine, [^{3}H]3-quinuclidinyl benzilate ([^{3}H]3-QNB), [^{3}H]4-N-methyl piperidinyl benzilate ([^{3}H]4-NMPB), [^{3}H]methyl scopolamine and [^{3}H]benzetimide and ^{3}H-labeled irreversible antagonists, e.g. [^{3}H]propyl benzilyl choline mustard ([^{3}H]PrBCM), were used to quantitate the muscarinic recognition sites (receptors) in the central and peripheral nervous systems[1,2] (and Refs. therein). These studies suggested that a homogenous population of muscarinic receptor sites bind the above antagonists with affinities in the nanomolar range. It is only recently that data on the regional heterogeneity of muscarinic antagonist binding was obtained in the mouse brain, where K_d values for 4-NMPB differ in different brain regions[3]. In the cerebral cortex and hippocampus, but not in the atria pirenzepine, a muscarinic antagonist was found to distinguish two classes of binding sites[4]. Using [^{3}H]4-NMPB two binding sites with different affinities were also shown in the rat and mouse pituitary (Avissar, Egozi and Sokolovsky, unpublished).

Kinetic studies on the binding of [^{3}H]3-QNB and [^{3}H]4-NMPB indicated that simple Langmuir isotherm which describes binding of those antagonists under equilibrium conditions may conceal a more complex reaction than a simple bimolecular association of the free receptor with the antagonist[3,5]. The observed rate constant for [^{3}H]3-QNB and [^{3}H]4-NMPB binding determined under pseudo-first-order conditions was not a linear but a hyperbolic function of the antagonist concentration[6]. One possible explanation of these results[3,5] is that the receptor–antagonist complex (RA) undergoes isomerization to form a more slowly dissociating complex (RA^+) according to equation [1]:

$$R + A \underset{k_{-1}}{\overset{k_1}{\rightleftharpoons}} RA \underset{k_{-2}}{\overset{k_2}{\rightleftharpoons}} RA^+ \quad [1]$$

where R and A are the receptor and antagonist, respectively. The equilibrium constants for the isomerization (k_{-2}/k_2) reaction for both [^{3}H]4-NMPB and [^{3}H]3-QNB were 0.15 in 50 mM phosphate buffer. It appears that the individual rate constants can be altered by changing the ionic composition of the medium. One may generalize the findings by stating that the ligand which can convert the receptor into a slowly dissociating complex is a good antagonist. Binding of antagonists does not show co-operativity in the sense that dissociation of RA^+ is not affected by agonists or antagonists. The binding of an antagonist to the receptor involves an increase in the entropy of the system.

Agonist binding

Until recently, agonist binding to the receptor was studied only by measuring the competition between a ^{3}H-labeled antagonist present at a constant concentration and varying concentrations of unlabeled agonists. Data from these experiments could be interpreted by assuming the existence of two populations of binding sites with different capacities and affinities[2], without assuming any co-operativity in agonist binding. In addition to the presence of 'high' and 'low' affinity agonist binding sites, Birdsall *et al.* reported that their non-linear least squares analysis revealed the existence of a 'super-high' affinity binding site in several brain regions (Ref. 2 and Refs therein).

A number of chemical modifying agents and treatments of membranes were found to alter the ratio of 'high' and 'low' affinity agonist binding sites in a given preparation. Effect of amino and thiol group specific reagents[7], e.g. NEM, pCMB, Cd^{2+}, revealed that agonist binding is more sensitive to modification of these groups than is antagonist binding, suggesting the presence of different subsites or conformers for agonist and antagonist binding. Study of the effects of NEM on the ratio of high and low affinity agonist binding sites gave the first suggestion that these binding sites are interconvertible and do not represent separate classes of 'isoreceptors' or receptors from different cell types. Receptors on a single cell type, N1E115, also show a high and a low affinity agonist binding[2]. Covalent modification of the receptor may take place *in vivo* by methylation, phosphorylation or thioltransferase reactions and may be the basis of short-term regulation of the receptor (cf. Fig. 1).

GTP and its analog have been extensively studied because they can convert high affinity agonist binding sites into low affinity binding sites without changing the total number[8]. It appears that hydrolysis of GTP which takes place during incubation with the membrane preparation is not an obligatory step required for the GTP effect since GDP and non-hydrolysable analogs of GTP can cause conversion of the receptor conformers similar to those caused by GTP. Thus, it is the binding of GTP, and not its energy of hydrolysis, which causes some conformational change in the receptor. Warming membranes to 50°C has similar effects to those produced by GTP, suggesting that some common conformational change may underlie the effects of heat and GTP[9].

GTP effects are regionally specific in the heart, cerebellum and medulla-pons but not to the same extent in the rest of the brain. In these tissues, muscarinic receptors mediate hyperpolarizing responses but it is not yet known whether the latter are associated with the GTP effects. It was shown that in the heart and in N1E115 neuroblastoma cells muscarinic agonists can inhibit the basal adenylate cyclase activity as well as the activation of adenylate cyclase by agonist-occupied

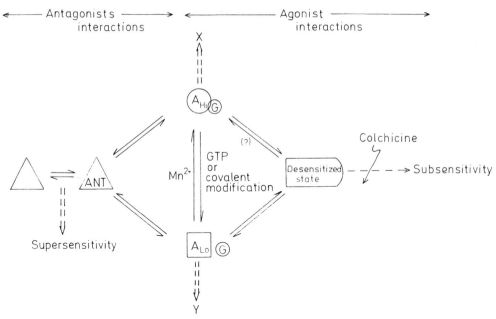

Fig. 1. Interactions of antagonists and agonists with the muscarinic receptor. The scheme summarizes the data described in the text with respect to receptor-antagonist (ANT) isomerization, shift in high (A_{Hi}) and low affinity (A_{Lo}) agonist binding states which are coupled or uncoupled to a nucleotide binding protein and desensitization. Some of the long term effects of occupancy with antagonist and agonist are indicated. Dashed arrows indicate processes which may involve, for example, internalization of receptors. Coupling of the agonist occupied receptors to targets X (e.g. nucleotide cyclases, sex hormone regulation of release) and Y (e.g. Ca^{2+}-channel, PI turnover or cGMP synthesis) are also indicated.

β-receptors. (see Ref. 11 for review). This inhibition of adenylate cyclase activity by muscarinic agonists requires Na^+, GTP and the hydrolysis of the latter. It is likely that the muscarinic receptor associates in the plane of the membrane with a nucleotide binding protein (N_i) of the adenylate cyclase complex[11] and thereby integrates the muscarinic and β-adrenergic responses at the cell membrane of the postsynaptic cell. Recent experiments (Hedlund and Bartfai, unpublished) show that addition of drugs which affect the voltage-dependent sodium channel, such as veratridine and tetrodotoxin, leads to the disappearance of high affinity agonist binding via blockade rather than interconversion. Treatments such as depolarization with high K^+, gramicidin or valinomycin or making the membranes leaky by freezing/thawing cycles lead to similar disappearance of high affinity agonist binding sites. These agents and treatments, unlike GTP, also change the affinity of antagonist binding[12].

The divalent transition metal ions Mn^{2+}, Co^{2+} and Ni^{2+} are the only agents presently known to convert low affinity agonist binding sites into high affinity binding sites[13]. This effect is unlikely to be due to complex formation with GTP, with which these ions form very stable (K_{MnGTP} $2.8 \cdot 10^{-6}$ M) complexes. An Antagonism between Ca^{2+} and Mn^{2+} also seems unlikely since the presence of 1 mM Ca^{2+} did not alter the effects of Mn^{2+}. It would appear that either Mn^{2+} mimics the action of a possible endogenous modulator or that it alters the hydrophobic interactions at the receptor site. However, Mn^{2+} may act through an activation of cGMP synthesis which is not mediated by a receptor[14]. This, in turn, may cause a cGMP-dependent modification (phosphorylation) or internalization of the receptor (a phenomenon of possible importance in 'desensitization').

The indirect measurement of agonist binding precludes independent estimation of the number of agonist and antagonist binding sites. The only answer that can be obtained is that all ^{3}H-labeled antagonist binding sites can be blocked by agonists whereas the opposite cannot be directly assessed. This leaves open the possibility that there are more agonist binding sites per receptor than antagonist binding site(s), assuming that the physiological response is elicited when more than one agonist is bound while it is blocked if at least one antagonist is bound. There are indirect indications of the possibility that more than one ligand may be bound to the receptor at the same time. First, kinetic studies on competition between agonist and ^{3}H-labeled antagonist showed that the first equilibrium $(k_{-1}/k_1)^{15}$ of equation [1] is apparently not affected by agonists such as oxotremorine and carbachol in concentrations which yield substantial inhibition of ^{3}H-labeled antagonist binding. If the sequential binding scheme is correct this may mean that agonists (B) bind with equal affinity to the free receptor (R) and the receptor–antagonist complex (RA).

If a ternary receptor–agonist–antagonist

$$R \rightleftharpoons RA \rightleftharpoons RA^+$$
$$\begin{array}{c} B \updownarrow \quad B \updownarrow \\ RB \rightleftharpoons RAB \\ B \updownarrow \\ RB_2 \end{array} \qquad [2]$$

complex (RAB) exists, then one should be able to determine this by using ^{3}H-labeled agonist and ^{3}H-labeled antagonist simultaneously, and indeed one of us recently has observed such a complex (Hedlund and Bartfai, unpublished results).

Direct binding studies of ^{3}H-labeled agonists have been carried out with [^{3}H]N-methyloxotremorine[2] and more recently with [^{3}H]cis-methyldioxolane[16], but in both cases only the high affinity sites were studied because the ratio of specific to nonspecific binding was very low (0.5–0.1). In the case of [^{3}H]pilocarpine, two plateaux were observed in the binding curve and the number of [^{3}H]pilocarpine binding sites as defined by competition with another agonist (oxotremorine 10^{-3} M) was higher than that of ^{3}H-labeled antagonist binding sites in the same preparation[17].

Regulation of muscarinic receptors

Responses mediated by muscarinic receptors may involve only a fraction of

TABLE I

Chemical treatments and *in vivo* manipulations which change the number and affinity of muscarinic receptors

Treatment	Tissue	Change in antagonist binding sites		Reference
		B_{max}	K_D	
Tetram	Hippocampus	54%	no change	20
Atropine	Dorsal hippocampus	80%	50% ↓ [a]	21
Septal lesion	Dorsal hippocampus	17%	no change	21
6OH-DA	Medulla-pons	17%	no change	22
Thyroidectomy	Heart	60%	no change	23
Barbiturate treatment	Midbrain	56%	no change	24
Amitriptyline	Medulla-pons			
	Hippocampus	25%	no change	25

[a] The apparent decrease in affinity may be due to residual atropine.

muscarinic receptor sites. Therefore, changes in the number of receptor sites, as determined by binding studies, may not necessarily reflect the change in the muscarinic responsivity. Another explanation for the discrepancy between muscarinic sensitivity and receptor number may be that the response involves a cascade of reactions beyond receptor occupancy. Nevertheless, it is clear that muscarinic receptors *per se* are subject to both short- and long-term regulation in certain tissues.

Short-term desensitization of the receptor may be an intrinsic part of the molecular mechanism of neurotransmitter-mediated events. Agonists in concentrations which result in occupancy of both high and low affinity sites, cause a rapid ($t_{\frac{1}{2}} < 4$ min) desensitization of the receptor-mediated increases in cGMP levels in N1E115 neuroblastoma cells[14,18]. Exposure to an agonist for such a short time does not change the number of antagonist binding sites. Studies on the effects of Mn^{2+} on carbamylcholine-desensitized cells suggest that a receptor-coupled Ca^{2+} channel is the desensitized part of the system which yields increased cGMP levels in response to agonist binding to the receptor. Na^+, K^+ and Mg^{2+} were without effect on the short-term desensitization of the cGMP response[18]. Histamine, the other neurotransmitter which raises cGMP levels in the same cells, did not influence desensitization of muscarinic receptors. This indicates that little or no coupling exists between the two receptors (H_1 and muscarinic) and that it is not 'feed-back' regulation by cGMP that stimulates its own synthesis[18].

Long-term incubation of neuroblastoma cells with muscarinic agonists cause a dose- and time-dependent loss of muscarinic receptor sites as measured by ^3H-labeled antagonists. Eighty per cent of the receptor sites were 'lost' in N1E115 cells on incubation for 9 h with carbamylcholine ($t_{\frac{1}{2}} = 3$ h)[19]. The ability to respond with increased cGMP levels to agonist binding falls faster than the number of antagonist binding sites, again suggesting that another component of the system is more easily desensitized than the recognition site carrying the polypeptide (receptor). When carbamylcholine is withdrawn, one finds a slow increase ($t_{\frac{1}{2}} = 8$ h) in ^3H-labeled antagonist binding, which depends on protein synthesis.

A number of *in vivo* treatments such as denervation or increased exposure to acetylcholine (e.g. through inhibition of acetylcholine esterase) were shown to change the number of antagonist binding sites (some selected examples are given in Table I). Recently, agonist binding was also studied in rats treated with estradiol and progesterone. These agents had a major effect both *in vivo* and *in vitro* on the distribution of receptors between high and low affinity agonist binding sites, and the affinity of the high affinity binding site increased tenfold. (Avissar and Sokolovsky, unpublished results.)

On the ionic mechanisms

Biochemical studies on changes in receptor number and affinity characterized the ligand-recognition site of the receptor but gave no information on the ionic mechanism of muscarinic action. We still do not know why muscarinic receptors with apparently identical recognition sites mediate hyperpolarization of heart cells and depolarization of Renshaw cells.

An obligatory role for Ca^{2+} was proven in postsynaptic muscarinic actions on smooth muscle cells[26] and on neuroblastoma (N1E115) cells[27]. Whether Ca^{2+} channels are directly coupled to receptors or the ominous increase in phosphatidyl inositol turnover[28] mediates changes in Ca^{2+} fluxes is not known. In parotid cells an increase in Ca^{2+}-dependent Na^+ fluxes was concomitant with receptor occupancy[29]. In the action of presynaptic muscarinic receptors, which regulate acetylcholine release by a feed-back mechanism (cf. Refs in Ref. 1) and have a somewhat different pharmacological profile from that of the postsynaptic receptors, no evidence could be found for changes in Ca^{2+} fluxes upon receptor occupancy while penetrating cGMP analogues mimicked the inhibitory effect of muscarinic agonists on the release.

Further work on the solubilization and purification of the receptor is clearly needed to achieve a functional reconstitution of the whole receptor unit thus allowing studies of its regulatory action on yet unidentified ion channels.

References

1 Heilbronn, E. and Bartfei, T. (1978) *Prog. Neurobiol.* 11, 171–188
2 Birdsall, N. J. M., Burgen, A. S. V. and Hulme, E. C. (1979) in *Recent Advances in Receptor Chemistry* (Gualtieri, F., Giannella, M. and Melchoirre, C., eds), pp. 71–96, Elsevier/North-Holland Biomedical Press
3 Kloog, Y., Egozi, Y. and Sokolovsky, M. (1979) *Mol. Pharmacol.* 15, 545–558
4 Hammer, R., Berrie, C. P., Birdsall, N. J. M., Burgen, A. S. V. and Hulme, E. C. (1980) *Nature (London)*, 283, 90–92
5 Galper, J. B. and Smith, J. W. (1978) *Proc. Natl Acad. Sci. U.S.A.* 75, 5831–5825
6 Järv, J., Hedlund, B. and Bartfai, T. (1979) *J. Biol. Chem.* 254, 5595–5598
7 Aronstam, R. S., Hoss, W. and Abood, L. G. (1977) *Eur. J. Pharmacol.* 46, 279–282
8 Sokolovsky, M., Gurwitz, D. and Galron, R. (1980) *Biochem. Biophys. Res. Commun.* 94, 487–492
9 Gurwitz, D. and Sokolovsky, M. (1980) *Biochem. Biophys. Res. Commun.* 94, 493–500
11 Rodbell, M. (1980) *Nature (London)*, 283, 17–22
12 Luqumani, Y. A., Bradford, H. F., Birdsall, N. J. M. and Hulme, E. C. (1979) *Nature (London)*, 277, 481–483
13 Gurwitz, D. and Sokolovsky, M. (1980) *Biochem. Biophys. Res. Commun.* 96, 1296–1305
14 El-Fakhany, E. and Richelson, E. (1980) *Proc. Natl Acad. Sci. U.S.A.* 77, 6897–6901
15 Järv, J., Hedlund, B. and Bartfai, T. (1980) *J. Biol. Chem.* 255, 2649–2651
16 Ehlert, F. J., Dumont, Y., Roeske, W. R. and Yamamura, H. I. (1980) *Life Sci.* 26, 961–967
17 Hedlund, B. and Bartfai, T. (1981) *Naunyn-Schmiedeberg's Arch. Pharmacol.* (in press)
18 El-Fakhany, E. and Richelson, E. (1980) *J. Neurochem.* 35, 941–948
19 Shifrin, G. S. and Klein, W. L. (1980) *J. Neurochem.* 34, 993–999
20 Gazit, H., Silman, I. and Dudai, Y. (1979) *Brain Res.* 174, 351–356
21 Westlind, A., Grynfarb, M., Hedlund, B., Bartfai, T. and Fuxe, K. (1981) *Brain Res.* (in press)
22 Gurwitz, D., Kloog, Y., Egozi, Y. and Sokolovsky, M. (1980) *Life Sci.* 26, 79–84
23 Sharma, V. K. and Banerjee, S. P. (1977) *J. Biol. Chem.* 252, 7444–7446
24 Nordberg, A., Wahlström, G. and Larsson, C. (1980) *Life Sci.* 26, 231–237
25 Rehavi, M., Ramot, O., Yavetz, B. and Sokolovsky, M. (1980) *Brain Res.* 194, 443–453
26 Triggle, D. J. (1979) in *Recent Advances in Receptor Chemistry* (Gualtieri, F., Giannella, M. and Melchoirre, C., eds), pp. 127–146, Elsevier/North-Holland Biomedical Press
27 Study, R. E., Breakefield, X. O., Bartfai, T. and Greengard, P. (1978) *Proc. Natl Acad. Sci. U.S.A.* 75, 6295–6299
28 Michell, R. H. (1975) *Biochem. Biophys. Acta*, 415, 81–147
29 Putney, J. W. Jr and Van De Walle, C. M. (1980) *J. Physiol. (London)*, 299, 521–531

Ligand occupation and the functional states of the nicotinic-cholinergic receptor

Palmer Taylor and Steven M. Sine

Division of Pharmacology, Department of Medicine, University of California, San Diego, La Jolla, CA 92093, U.S.A.

Simultaneous measurements of receptor occupation and the change in ion permeability elicited by the ligands enable one to define the linkage between agonist association and activation of the ion channel. The nicotinic receptor behaves effectively as a co-operative dimer. Two agonist molecules are required for activation while a single bound antagonist is sufficient to block the response of the receptor oligomer. The two agonist binding sites on the oligomer do not show precise functional equivalence as might be anticipated from the arrangement of subunits of this protein in the membrane.

Introduction

The availability of selective peptide toxins that act on the nicotinic-cholinergic receptor and an abundant tissue source for the receptor itself have facilitated a relatively detailed characterization of the structure and ligand binding properties of this membrane protein. These subjects have been considered in a number of recent reviews[1,2]. Also, recent electrophysiological studies have defined the primary events associated with the opening and closing of individual receptor-linked channels[3]. Thus, with the structural definition and biophysical experimentation on this receptor developing to an advanced stage, it would seem topical to consider the relationship between the recognition and functional capacities of the receptor. Underlying this linkage is the basis of pharmacological selectivity of agonists, partial agonists and antagonists. In this review, we will attempt to provide a simplifying conceptual framework for analysing the predominant functional states of the receptor consistent with its molecular structure.

To approach the question of the relationship between occupation and the functional response, simultaneous measures of both parameters are required. At present, two systems seem suited for this purpose. The first is the isolated and sealed vesicle isolated from homogenates of *Torpedo* sp. electric organs (see Refs 1, 2 and 4). This system carries the advantages that measurements are made on the same receptor in which structural characterization is most complete and the system can be studied in suspension which permits measurements of permeability and occupation in a time frame approaching several milliseconds[4]. The second system is cultured muscle cells which when grown in monolayer allow for equivalent exposure of agonists to surface receptors[5]. In a clonal cell line, such as the BC3H-1 cells to be considered, each cell is the daughter of a single progenitor and permeability changes can be monitored in cells of comparatively uniform size and shape. The cell line also carries the advantages that measurements can be conducted on mammalian receptors in intact cells and that flux in the appropriate inward direction is ascertained for the major current-carrying ion involved in agonist-elicited depolarization of the membrane, Na^+. For analysis of permeability by ion fluxes, it is important not to violate initial rate conditions for the entire population of cells or organelles. Thus, one strives to achieve a relatively narrow size distribution of enclosed volumes. The relatively small surface-to-internal volume ratio of intact cells compared to membrane vesicles also enables one to carry out experiments over a more extended time frame. Desensitization can be minimized by working at 3°, but desensitization steps occurring in the subsecond time frame will not be detected with these flux assays. To ensure that permeability is not influenced by changes in membrane potential during measurements of unidirectional flux, potential is adjusted to near zero by balancing external and internal Na^+ and K^+.

There is now considerable evidence documenting that the cholinergic receptor is a pentamer composed of four different subunits in the stoichiometric ratio $\alpha_2, \beta, \gamma, \delta$[1]. The two α-subunits each carry a single recognition site which exhibits mutually exclusive binding for agonists, reversible antagonists and the near-irreversible peptide antagonists, the α-toxins. The precise functional role of the other subunits is not known but it is likely that some or all of the subunits form the outer shell of the channel which controls ion permeability. Receptor activation, both in the intact endplate[3] and in isolated cells and vesicles[4–6], occurs over a narrow concentration range, and exhibits positive co-operativity. Thus, occupation of more than a single site is required for the linked opening of a channel and one might envisage that a concerted transition between the subunits is required for this activation step.

Occupation and activation by agonists

Under conditions where we are able to eliminate a certain fraction of binding sites, let us consider how the residual permeability response will be affected. Since the α-toxins bind with high affinity to the sites on the two α-subunits and for the purposes of these experiments the binding is irreversible, they offer an ideal means for fractionally inactivating the surface binding sites on the intact cell. Moreover, since the association rate of α-toxin exhibits bimolecularity, no selectivity for either of the two sites or co-operativity in binding is evident[5,6]. Accordingly, with a 50% overall occupation of the sites the species of receptor–toxin complexes should exhibit a binomial distribution where 25% of the receptors are totally unoccupied, 25% are fully occupied by 2 α-toxin molecules, and the remaining 50% are essentially 'hybrid' species carrying a vacant site and one bound α-toxin molecule at the other site. Upon addition of agonist, should the hybrids be non-functional, overall occupation by α-toxin of 50% of the sites leads to a residual response of 25% (Fig. 1A).

The more general equations for the relationship between prior α-toxin occupation and the residual response are given in Fig. 1B. Experimentally[6], we find that the relationship between α-toxin occupation, y, and the fractional permeability k_G/k_{Go} is best described by a parabolic function of the form

$$k_G/k_{Go} = (1 - y)^2. \qquad (1)$$

Thus, at least two bound agonist molecules

are required for receptor activation and hybrid species carrying a bound α-toxin molecule and the agonist (i.e. carbamylcholine) remain mute with respect to ion permeability.

Should this relationship hold, two corroborating observations are necessary to complete the argument. First, since only the doubly-unoccupied species will respond to subsequent agonist exposure with a change in permeability, fractional titration of sites with α-toxin should not alter concentration dependence for activation of the residual active receptors. We observe that the positive co-operativity for activation ($n_H = 1.6-1.7$) is not affected by prior α-toxin occupation[6]. Second, with a concerted interaction between subunits involved in activation, we would anticipate that prior occupation by α-toxin would influence carbamylcholine occupation of the neighbor of paired sites in the dimer. Thus, upon prior titration with α-toxin, the hybrid species will begin to predominate over the doubly-unoccupied species by the ratio $2y(1-y)/(1-y)^2$ and the positive co-operativity for occupation by the agonist should diminish. In fact, not only is the Hill coefficient (n_H) for carbamylcholine occupation diminished but as y increases, n_H goes through unity and approaches a limiting value of 0.65 (Ref. 6). This observation holds for association with the low affinity states (which measures binding to the activatable and active states of the receptor) as well as for association at

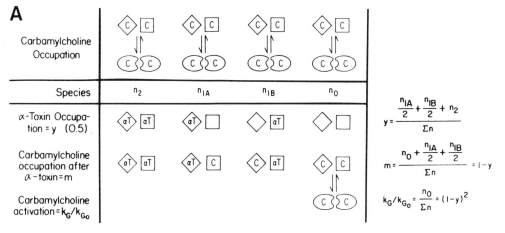

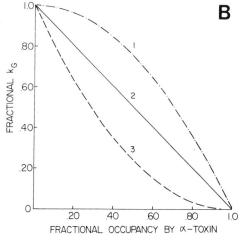

Fig. 1. (A) The relationship between prior α-toxin (αT) occupation and carbamylcholine (C) occupation and activation of an oligomeric receptor containing two binding sites. (B) Relationships between the fractional permeability k_G/k_{Go}, and prior α-toxin occupation (y), for a receptor containing two binding sites. (1) Hybrid species containing bound α-toxin and agonist on each oligomer are fully active, $k_G/k_{Go} = (1 - y^2)$. (2) Hybrid species display one half of the permeability response to applied carbamylcholine as the doubly-unoccupied species, $k_G/k_{Go} = 1 - y$. (3) Hybrid species are inactive, $k_G/k_{Go} = (1 - y)^2$.

equilibrium (which also includes binding to the desensitized state of the receptor). The fact that a limiting Hill coefficient of less than unity is achieved, indicates that the two α-subunits are not functionally equivalent and the concerted transition is superimposed on this intrinsic binding inequivalence of the two α-subunits. We shall return to this point later.

Association of antagonists with the receptor and functional antagonism

Antagonists are found to exhibit Hill coefficients of less than unity for their association with the receptor[5,7-9]. This might be expected considering the above described agonist behavior where inequivalent binding properties are uncovered when the concerted transitions between states are abolished. Classical antagonists, of course, do not promote the transition associated with activation or channel opening and show little or no propensity for driving the receptor into its desensitized state[8]. Hill coefficients less than unity for antagonists could be due to three possibilities. The least probable is true negative co-operativity where antagonist binding to one of the two sites diminishes the affinity of the neighboring site for this ligand. This can be ruled out by the observation that prior occupation by α-toxin does not alter the concentration dependence of antagonist binding to the residual sites[6]. In the negative co-operativity model, convergence to a Hill coefficient of 1.0 would be expected as hybrid species are formed. The other two possibilities for the low Hill coefficient involve the nonequivalence of binding sites and here we can develop two limiting cases: either the two nonequivalent sites, A and B, are confined to a single oligomer (i.e. AB oligomers), or two types of receptors which contain identically paired subunits are present (AA and BB oligomers). In the event that the two types of receptors (AA and BB) were present in near-equal populations, binding experiments alone would not distinguish between these two possibilities. In both cases

$$\frac{\text{fractional}}{\text{occupation}} = 0.5(X_A) + 0.5(X_B) \quad (2)$$

$$= 0.5\left(\frac{L}{L + K_A}\right) + 0.5\left(\frac{L}{L + K_B}\right) \quad (3)$$

where L is the ligand concentration, X_A and X_B are the fractional occupations of the A and B sites, respectively, and K_A and K_B are the respective dissociation constants.

It is to be expected that reversible antagonists, like α-toxin, will block an agonist-elicited response by binding to a single site. Then, if the binding sites are confined to a single oligomer

$$k_G/k_{Go} = (1 - X_A)(1 - X_B) \quad (4)$$

$$= \left(\frac{K_A}{L + K_A}\right)\left(\frac{K_B}{L + K_B}\right). \quad (5)$$

If the non-equivalent sites exist on separate oligomers each containing identically paired subunits, then

$$k_G/k_{Go} = 0.5(1 - X_A)^2 + 0.5(1 - X_B)^2 \quad (6)$$

$$= 0.5\left(\frac{K_A}{L + K_A}\right)^2 + 0.5\left(\frac{K_B}{L + K_B}\right)^2 \quad (7)$$

When $K_A \rightarrow K_B$, equations 5 and 7 converge, whereas when K_A and K_B differ, the overall functions differ substantially. Shown in Fig. 2 are the corresponding functions for binding and functional antagonism when $K_B = 4K_A$ and $K_B = 50K_A$. In the latter case we should be able to distinguish between mechanisms. Data for the association of five classical nicotinic antagonists reveal Hill coefficients of less than one (Table I) and the binding curves can all be fitted to a two-site model in which there are equal populations of sites with differing dissociation constants. Within this series of antagonists K_B/K_A ranges between 4 and 89. Thus, by obtaining dissociation constants from the occupation curves (equation 3) one can compare the concentration

TABLE I. Parameters for antagonist occupation of receptors on BC3H-1 cells: inhibition of the permeability change elicited by carbamylcholine

Antagonist	K_P, M[a]	n_{Hp}[a]	K_A, M[b]	K_B, M[b]	K_B/K_A	K_{ant}, M[c]	n_{Ha}[c]	$\dfrac{K_P}{K_{ant}}$
Alcuronium	4.18×10^{-8}	0.87 ± 0.03	2.14×10^{-8}	1.68×10^{-8}	4.1	1.28×10^{-8}	0.99 ± 0.02	3.3
Pancuronium	2.33×10^{-8}	0.86 ± 0.02	9.11×10^{-9}	6.93×10^{-8}	7.6	7.38×10^{-9}	1.16 ± 0.07	3.2
AH8165	6.01×10^{-7}	0.78 ± 0.01	1.83×10^{-7}	1.84×10^{-6}	10.3	2.08×10^{-7}	1.08 ± 0.03	2.9
Gallamine	1.46×10^{-5}	0.70 ± 0.03	3.70×10^{-6}	5.50×10^{-5}	14.8	3.68×10^{-6}	1.00 ± 0.06	4.0
Dimethyl d-tubocurarine	3.07×10^{-6}	0.51 ± 0.03	3.09×10^{-7}	2.75×10^{-5}	89.0	4.69×10^{-7}	0.85 ± 0.05	6.9

[a] K_P is the concentration of antagonist at 50% occupation and n_{Hp} is the associated Hill coefficient. Occupation was ascertained by the antagonists' capacity to inhibit the initial rate of α-toxin association[7].
[b] K_A and K_B are the high and low affinity intrinsic dissociation constants resulting from the fit of experimental data to equation 3.
[c] K_{ant} is the concentration of antagonist which decreases the permeability increase elicited by 30 μM carbamylcholine by 50% and n_{Ha} is the associated Hill coefficient (cf. Ref. 7).

dependence for functional antagonism with the predictions of equations 5 and 7. Our experimental observations in the mammalian cells clearly show a close correspondence with equation 5 or the limiting case where the two sites are confined to a single oligomer[7].

Another approach allows one to corroborate this model. We have mentioned previously that cobra α-toxin association rates do not show selectivity between the sites on the α-subunits. However, if cobra α-toxin association were allowed to occur in the presence of an antagonist (such as dimethyl-d-tubocurarine) which is present in concentrations sufficient to occupy primarily the high affinity site, the toxin would be directed to the low affinity or B sites. Subsequent washing of the cell surface removes the dimethyl-d-tubocurarine with α-toxin being retained on the B sites. It can then be demonstrated that dimethyl-d-tubocurarine binding to the vacant sites follows the behavior of binding to a single class of sites of high affinity. A Hill coefficient approaching 1.0 and a dissociation constant approaching K_A are found[7]. Thus, now possessing a means for selectively directing α-toxin to one of the two sites, let us return to the relationship

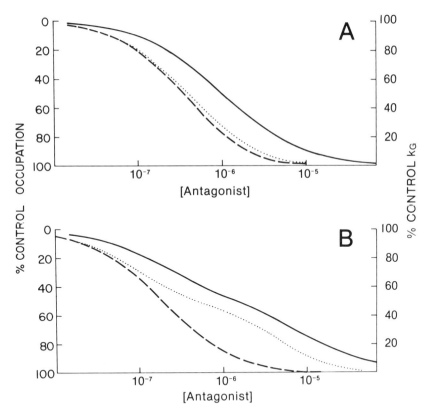

Fig. 2. Concentration dependencies for occupation and functional antagonism using a two-site description of antagonist binding where the sites are present in equal populations. The solid lines in each panel depict the occupation curves. The corresponding dashed lines represent inhibition of the agonist-elicited permeability, k_G, for AB oligomers where non-equivalent sites are confined to a single oligomer (equation 5). The dotted lines represent inhibition of agonist-elicited permeability where the sites exist on two distinct oligomers and the sites are identically paired on each oligomer (AA and BB oligomers) (equation 7). In panel A antagonist affinities for the A and B sites differ by a factor of 4 ($K_A = 5 \times 10^{-7}$, $K_B = 2 \times 10^{-6}$M) while in panel B they differ by 50 fold ($K_A = 2 \times 10^{-7}$, $K_B = 1 \times 10^{-5}$M).

between fractional permeability (k_G/k_{Go}) and α-toxin occupation, y.

If the two sites are confined to a single oligomer (AB oligomers), then

$$k_G/k_{Go} = (1 - y_A)(1 - y_B). \quad (8)$$

while if two different oligomers with identically paired subunits (AA and BB) exist:

$$k_G/k_{Go} = 0.5 (1 - y_A)^2 + 0.5(1 - y_B)^2. \quad (9)$$

Since $(1 - y_A)(1 - y_B) < (1 - y)^2 < 0.5(1 - y_A)^2 + 0.5(1 - y_B)^2$, a comparison of the fractional permeability following selective and non-selective direction of α-toxin to its sites should distinguish between limiting cases. We find that a greater reduction in permeability results with selective direction of α-toxin rather than random direction, which is again consistent with the non-equivalent sites being confined to one oligomer[7]. Intuitively, in the AB oligomer model we would expect the greater fractional reduction of permeability when α-toxin sites are labeled in the presence of a reversible antagonist, since the abundance of hybrid species would exceed that predicted by a binomial distribution.

While the data are consistent with the major population of receptors existing as AB oligomers rather than AA and BB pairs, it becomes more difficult to distinguish this limiting model from more complex arrangements of subunits. For example, three or more distinct oligomers could arise through associations of the subunits (AA, AB, BB). For the $\alpha_2\beta\gamma\delta$ composition, such arrangements require either differences in subunit components within the individual oligomers or permutations in the subunit arrangements[11]. While more complex models introduce additional free parameters and hence could provide a closer correspondence with the experimental data, experiments in this system lack the precision to distinguish the small quantitative differences between complex models. The AB oligomer scheme is defined simply by a single receptor species while all other arrangements dictate that multiple oligomeric receptor species are present.

Thus, this rather straightforward approach reveals that the nicotinic receptor can be described in terms of a functionally asymmetric oligomer in which the two sites within the oligomer do not exhibit equal binding affinities in the case of both agonists and reversible antagonists. For antagonist association this is reflected in Hill coefficients of less than 1.0. Agonists, however, initiate state transitions both for activation and desensitization. Positive co-operativity is evident and thus at least two agonist molecules are required to effect a concerted transition to the activated (open channel) and to the desensitized state. Analyses of both the binding and state functions for desensitization would suggest that a concerted or symmetry driven mechanism best describes these transitions. Receptor hybrids that form containing bound α-toxin and agonist or reversible antagonists and agonists do not appear to convert to the open channel state nor do they show a positively co-operative transition to the desensitized state. It is only when the hybrid species predominates and the concerted transition is unable to occur, that the inequivalence in the two agonist sites is revealed.

Structural implications

Even though on the basis of available N-terminal sequences the two α-subunits appear chemically identical[10], their functional inequivalence is not unexpected. Non-symmetrical arrangements and functional inequivalence have been shown for simple dimeric enzymes containing chemically identical subunits. With the receptor additional constraints are imposed from the addition of the β, γ and δ subunits. Since most and possibly all of the subunits traverse the membrane[1] and all display considerable sequence homology[10], it is likely that similar segments in the linear sequence of each subunit form the presumed α-helical domains that traverse the membrane bilayer. Arranging the subunits as in Fig. 3 necessitates that the inter-subunit contacts for the two α-subunits will not be identical. Accordingly, it is not possible to place a two-fold axis of symmetry perpendicular to the membrane. Thus, a structural basis exists for the functional inequivalence as well as for differences in sulfhydryl reactivity[12,13] of the α-subunits.

Finally, a comparison of the concentration dependencies for antagonist occupation and functional antagonism reveals certain salient features in the analysis of dose–response curves (Fig. 2). First the concentration dependencies of occupation and antagonism are not identical as we can see in the two extremes. For antagonism of responses elicited at low agonist occupation, when $K_A \ll K_B$, $K_{ant} = K_A$, whereas when $K_A \to K_B$, then

$$K_{ant} = \frac{\sqrt{K_A K_B}}{1 + \sqrt{2}} \simeq \frac{K_A}{2.414} \quad (10)$$

Secondly, Hill coefficients for the concentration dependencies of functional antagonism are predicted to be larger than the corresponding values for receptor occupation. For functional antagonism, when K_A and K_B differ, $n_H = 1.0$, whereas in the limit of $K_A \to K_B$, $n_H \simeq 1.2$ In the pharmacological quantitation of competitive antagonism, a null method or Schild plot[14] is typically employed to determine the dissociation constant for the antagonist. For oligomeric receptors such as in the situation above, an essentially parallel shift of the dose–response curve will still be achieved in the presence of competitive antagonists yet the dissociation constant for functional antagonism calculated from the ratio of agonist concentrations will not necessarily equal the apparent dissociation constant for occupation of the receptor by the antagonist. Hence, for the various receptor types, an understanding of the mechanism of antagonism is needed to relate quantitatively the dissociation constant obtained from either a null-method or antagonism measured at low agonist occupation to the true dissociation constant(s).

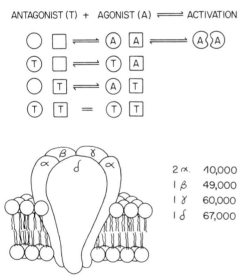

Fig. 3. Description of the various species of receptor capable of antagonist (T) and agonist (A) occupation and activation. The receptor is depicted as a dimer of binding sites in which a concerted transition is required for activation and the two sites do not show precise equivalence. In the lower portion, a plausible structural organization of subunits, α, β, γ, δ, is shown which would allow for the nonequivalence of both agonist and antagonist binding in each oligomer, the positive co-operativity and presumed concerted interaction required for receptor activation and desensitization. See text for details. The ligand binding sites are found on the α-subunits and all five subunits form the perimeter of the ion channel.

Reading list

1 Karlin, A. (1980) in *The Cell Surface and Neuronal Function* (Poste, G., Nicolson, G. L. and Cotman, C. W., eds), Vol. 5, pp. 191–260, Elsevier/North Holland, New York
2 Giraudat, J. and Changeux, J. P. (1980) *Trends Pharmacol. Sci.* 1, 198–202
3 Steinbach, J. H. (1980) in *The Cell Surface and Neuronal Function* (Poste, G., Nicolson, G. L. and Cotman. C. W., eds), Vol. 5, pp. 119–156, Elsevier/North Holland, New York
4 Neubig, R. and Cohen, J. B. (1980) *Biochemistry* 19, 2770–2779

5 Sine, S. and Taylor, P. (1979) *J. Biol. Chem.* 254, 3315–3325
6 Sine, S. and Taylor, P. (1980) *J. Biol. Chem.* 255, 10144–10156
7 Sine, S. and Taylor, P. (1981) *J. Biol. Chem.* 256, 6692–6699
8 Weiland, G. and Taylor, P. (1979) *Mol. Pharmacol.* 15, 197–212
9 Neubig, R. R. and Cohen, J. B. (1979) *Biochemistry* 18, 5465–5475
10 Raftery, M. A., Hunkapiller, M. W., Strader, C. D. and Hood, L. E. (1980) *Science* 208, 1454–1456
11 Taylor, P. and Sine, S. (1981) in *Chemical Transmission: 75 years*, Second Nobel Conference, pp. 347–359, Academic Press, London
12 Damle, V. N. and Karlin, A. (1978) *Biochemistry* 17, 2035–2049
13 Wolosin, J. M., Lyddiat, A., Dolly, J. O. and Barnard, E. A. (1980) *Eur. J. Biochem.* 109, 495–505
14 Schild, H. O. (1949) *Br. J. Pharmacol.* 4, 227–230

Recent developments in histamine H₂-antagonists

R. T. Brittain, D. Jack, and B. J. Price

Glaxo Group Research Ltd, Ware Division, Ware, Herts, U.K.

Classification of histamine receptors and a physiological role for histamine

Although Ash and Schild[1] showed that there is more than one type of histamine receptor and proposed that those specifically blocked by the then known histamine antagonists, such as mepyramine, be termed H_1-receptors, it was the definitive work of Black *et al.*[2] which established that the pharmacological effects of histamines are mediated by two distinctively different receptors which they called histamine H_1- and H_2-receptors. This classification was based on the different sensitivities of histamine receptors in a variety of preparations to the agonistic actions of a few close analogues of histamine and on their discovery of selective H_2-antagonists. The latter were substituted imidazoles, burimamide (**I**) being followed by metiamide (**II**) and cimetidine (**III**).

Responses mediated by histamine H_1-receptors include contraction of bronchial and intestinal smooth muscle; their biochemical mechanism is unknown. Responses mediated by H_2-receptors include increase in the frequency and force of contraction of cardiac muscle, relaxation of uterine smooth muscle and secretion of gastric acid, all of which are consequences of stimulation of adenylate cyclase by H_2-agonists whose action is akin to that of β-adrenoceptor stimulants. Vascular smooth muscle contains H_1- and H_2- receptors both of which mediate vasodilatation.

Burimamide is a historic compound because it was found to inhibit acid secretion in animals and man induced by infusion of histamine or pentagastrin, or by ingestion of food. Thus, for the first time Black and his colleagues showed histamine to be the ultimate extracellular physiological mediator of acid secretion by the parietal cells in the gastric pits. Burimamide itself is not a useful medicine because it is poorly absorbed from the alimentary tract. The more potent, metiamide, is an orally active inhibitor of acid secretion and was found to induce healing of duodenal and gastric ulcers. Regrettably, its use had to be discontinued because it caused agranulocytosis in some patients. It was superseded by cimetidine which has been extensively used because of its great therapeutic efficacy in peptic ulcer disease and other conditions in which inhibition of acid secretion is desirable.

Cimetidine is not without its limitations. Because it is short-acting it requires a frequent dosing schedule in man and, more fundamentally, its specificity of action is poor. Cimetidine has anti-adrenogenic activity which can lead to gynaecomastia in man and it inhibits the cytochrome P450 mixed function oxygenase metabolising enzyme systems in the liver[3], an action which potentiates the effects of drugs such as warfarin or valium administered concur-

Burimamide (**I**): imidazole–CH₂CH₂CH₂CH₂NH–C(=S)–NHMe

Metiamide (**II**): 5-Me-imidazole–CH₂SCH₂CH₂NH–C(=S)–NHMe

Cimetidine (**III**): 5-Me-imidazole–CH₂SCH₂CH₂NH–C(=NCN)–NHMe

rently with cimetidine because they are inactivated by this enzyme system. Cimetidine also causes confusional states in some elderly patients by an unknown mechanism. Clearly, an improved H$_2$-antagonist is desirable and this paper describes work directed towards this objective. Much of it was carried out in the Ware Division, Glaxo Group Research Ltd, and we are grateful to our colleagues for permission to use some of their results. Fuller details are contained in the patent literature and more will be published in due course by the various teams involved.

Experimental determination of histamine H$_2$-antagonism

Histamine H$_2$-antagonism in a drug is most conveniently determined *in vitro* using the chronotropic response of guinea-pig right atrium or the relaxation of rat uterus caused by histamine. The nature of the antagonism[4] is determined and quantified from the dose-dependant displacements of the histamine concentration–effect curves. Specificity of action of the antagonists is investigated using preparations such as guinea-pig ileum, which contain only H$_1$-receptors, and other preparations responsive to other agonists such as isoprenaline, a typical β-adrenoceptor stimulant, and bethanecol, a cholinergic agent.

Inhibition of acid secretion is most easily determined using a perfused stomach preparation in the anaesthetized rat[5] in which the effect of intravenously administered drug on histamine- or pentagastrin-induced gastric acid secretion is determined. Oral activity and the duration of action are measured using conscious dogs with Heidenhain pouches in which it is possible to study drug effects on acid secretion induced by histamine, bethanecol or pentagastrin[6]. Conscious dogs with gastric fistulas are used to study secretory responses to test meals[7].

Non-imidazole histamine H$_2$-antagonists

A common feature of the H$_2$-antagonists discovered by Black and his colleagues was an imidazole ring. That an imidazole, or a similar basic heterocyclic ring, might not be necessary for H$_2$-blocking activity was investigated by replacing the imidazole moiety by an alternative aromatic ring system, including furan, thiophene and benzene. We soon found that for H$_2$-blocking activity it was necessary to incorporate a basic substituent in the non-basic ring. The results for the furan series were particularly encouraging, the thiourea (**IV**) and the cyanoguanidine (**V**) being only a little less active than their imidazole analogues, metiamide and cimetidine. The nitro-ethene derivative (**VI**) was especially interesting being at least five times more active than cimetidine and substantially more active than its imidazole analogue (**VII**) as an inhibitor of histamine induced acid secretion in the anaesthetised rat. These few results make it clear that structure–activity relationships in H$_2$-antagonists vary with the nature of the aromatic centre. The ethene (**VI**), now known as ranitidine, is considered in greater detail later.

The investigation of the effect of methyl-substitution in the furan ring proved to be interesting. 5-Methyl substitution in the imidazole series confers increased potency and so we thought that the 3-methyl furan analogues might be more active than their 4-methyl-isomers (**VIII**) but were surprised when the 3-methyl derivative (**IX**) proved inactive whereas the 4-isomer (**X**) was a highly potent antagonist.

The 2,5-substitution pattern in our original furan derivatives arose purely from chemical considerations since 2-substituted furans readily take part in the Mannich reaction and the products are 2,5-disubstituted. This proved to be by far the optimum arrangement since none of the other five disubstitutions (compounds **XI–XV**) possessed significant antisecretory activity.

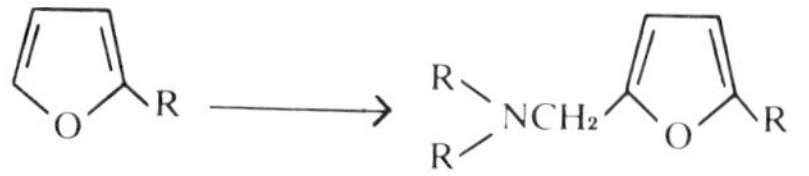

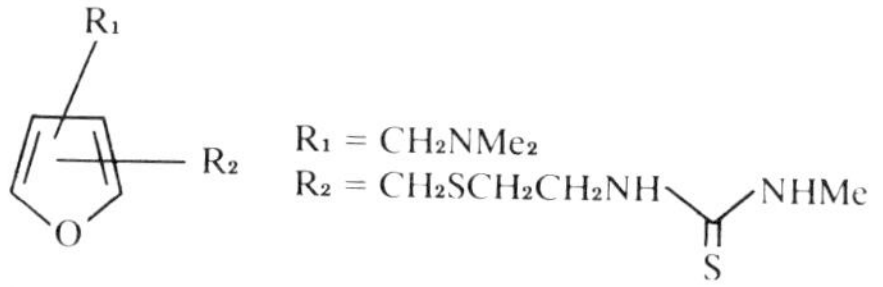

$R_1 = CH_2NMe_2$
$R_2 = CH_2SCH_2CH_2NH-C(=S)-NHMe$

The replacement of the furan by another non-basic ring system appropriately substituted with a dimethylaminomethyl group was of interest and the thiophene derivative (**XVI**) was found to be less active than the corresponding furan and the benzene derivative (**XVII**) still less active. Thus, increasing lipophilicity was associated with decreasing histamine H_2-blocking activity in this series.

Pharmacological and clinical studies with ranitidine

Ranitidine, $0.1–1\ \mu g\ ml^{-1}$, competitively antagonized the action of histamine on the isolated guinea-pig atrium and rat uterus, preparations known to possess H_2-receptors. In these experiments ranitidine was about five times more potent than cimetidine. The blocking action of ranitidine was highly specific for H_2-receptors since the much higher dose, $30\ \mu g\ ml^{-1}$, had no effect on β-adrenoceptors in guinea-pig atria, or on H_1-receptors or

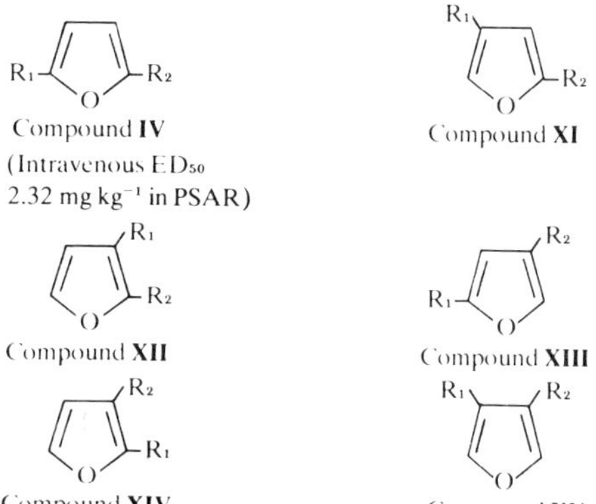

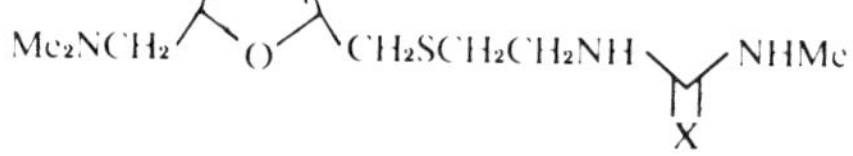

Compound **IV** (Intravenous ED_{50} 2.32 mg kg^{-1} in PSAR)

Compound **XI**

Compound **XII**

Compound **XIII**

Compound **XIV**

Compound **XV**

Intravenous ED_{50} (mg kg^{-1}) in inhibiting histamine-induced acid secretion in the perfused stomach preparation of the anaesthetized rat (PSAR)

Compound **IV**	X = S	2.32
Compound **V**	X = N–CN	1.39
Compound **VI** (Ranitidine)	X = CH–NO$_2$	0.13

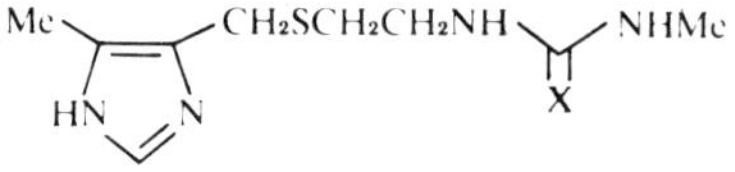

VIII

Compound **II** (Metiamide)	X = S	0.52
Compound **III** (Cimetidine)	X = N–CN	0.73
Compound **VII**	X = CH–NO$_2$	1.75

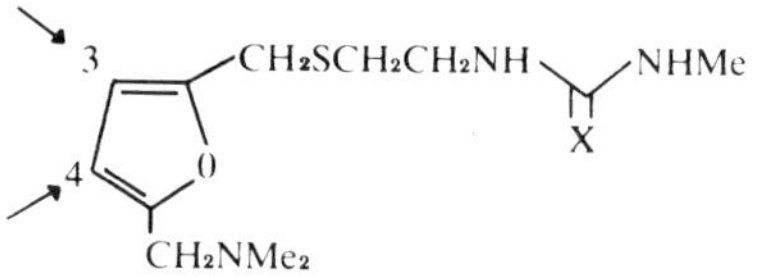

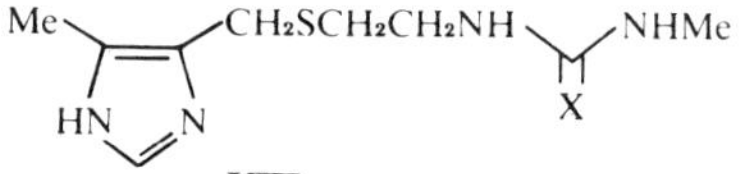

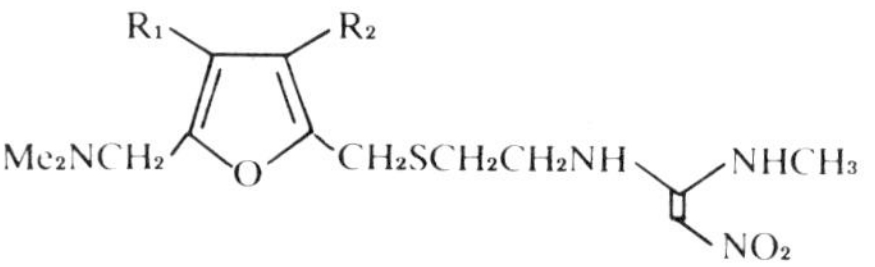

Intravenous ED_{50} (mg kg^{-1}) in PSAR

Compound **IX**	R_1 = H, R_2 = Me	>10
Compound **X**	R_1 = Me, R_2 = H	0.25

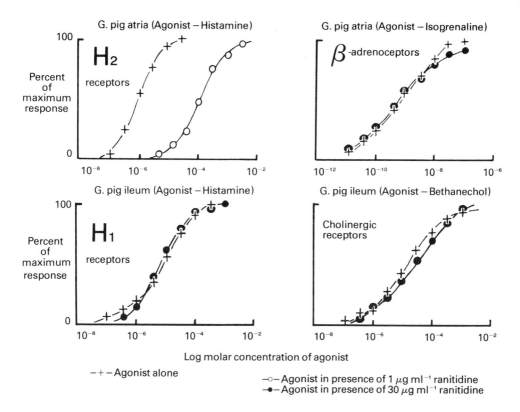

Fig. 1. Effects of ranitidine against histamine, isoprenaline and bethanechol induced responses on isolated tissues.

cholinergic receptors in guinea-pig ileum. Representative results are shown in Fig. 1.

Ranitidine potently inhibited histamine-induced acid secretion in the conscious Heidenhain-pouched dog, the oral ED_{50} values for ranitidine and cimetidine being 0.23 and 0.96 mg kg^{-1} respectively. In these experiments equi-effective doses of the drugs had similar onsets of action but with ranitidine, appreciable anti-secretory activity was evident after 5 h, whereas recovery was complete after 4½ h with cimetidine.

Conscious dogs with well-established gastric fistulas were used to study the effects of the drugs on the secretory response to a test meal, a procedure which is considered to be the most relevant for the clinical situation. Intravenously infused ranitidine, 0.03–0.3 mg kg^{-1} h^{-1}, and cimetidine, 0.3–3.0 mg kg^{-1} h^{-1} both caused dose-dependant inhibitions of acid secretion. As shown in Fig. 2, ranitidine was about ten times more active than cimetidine. The inhibition of gastric acid secretion caused by ranitidine is not a consequence of reduced mucosal blood flow[6] but results entirely from specific blockade of H_2-receptors on the parietal cells.

Since, as already explained, cimetidine has relatively poor specificity of action, it was important to subject ranitidine to appropriate additional tests to see if its action was more specific. In brief, ranitidine, administered over prolonged periods to rats had no detectable anti-androgenic activity[8] nor did it inhibit the cytochrome P450 enzyme system in rat liver[9]. Ranitidine is, therefore, more selectively acting than cimetidine.

Ranitidine is quite well absorbed from the gastro-intestinal tract in animals and man (bioavailability about 50%) and is excreted mainly unchanged in the urine.

The urinary metabolites in man represent about 2% of the oral dose and are the N-oxide and sulphoxide of ranitidine and N-desmethyl ranitidine. In autoradiographic studies using labelled drug, no radioactivity was detectable in the CNS of animals and so side-effects are not likely to occur with ranitidine.

Detailed toxicological and reproductive studies on ranitidine have not revealed drug-related effects which would limit its clinical use. Indeed, its potency, freedom from toxicity and relatively long duration of action, allows the single oral dose of the drug in man to be 150 mg which controls acid secretion for up to 12 h. The drug has been found to be effective in the treatment of acute ulcers when given twice daily, most duodenal and gastric ulcers being healed within 4–6 weeks. Its great selectivity of action has been confirmed in man and no serious side effects have been reported in the first 2000 patients at the therapeutic regimen or in more than 100 treated continuously for more than one year at the maintenance dosage, 150 mg at night. Clinical trials are continuing.

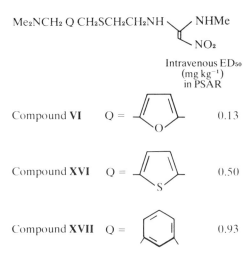

Future directions in research

Undoubtedly further potent, selective H_2-antagonists will be found and already cimetidine analogues incorporating thiazole (**XVIII**) or oxazole (**XIX**) rings have been described. Tiotidine (**XVIII**) is about five times more active than cimetidine and has a relatively slow onset but a prolonged action in man[10]. Clinical trials on it were stopped when it was found to cause carcinoma in the antrum of the

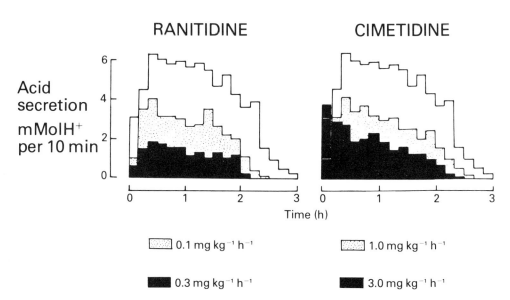

Fig. 2. Effects of ranitidine and cimetidine on the secretory response to a test meal in the conscious dog with a gastric fistula.

stomach of the rat. The oxazole[11] may be more active than cimetidine but information on this compound is extremely limited.

Other new compounds are imidazoles. Etintidine (**XX**) a propargyl analogue of cimetidine seems similar to that drug[12]. Oxmetidine (**XXI**), a benzyl-pyrimidone derivate is more novel and is about eight times and two times more active than cimetidine after intravenous and oral use respectively in man[13] but is no longer acting than cimetidine. On the present evidence ranitidine has advantages over cimetidine because it lacks the side effects associated with the latter drug and is more convenient to use. If ranitidine remains unflawed what further progress is desirable or possible in an H_2-antagonist? The answer appears to be very little, other than a controlled prolonged selective action, which allows once daily therapeutic dosage.

Reading list

1 Ash, A. S. F. and Schild, H. O. (1966) *Br. J. Pharmac.* 27, 427–439
2 Black, J. W., Duncan, W. A. M., Durrant, C. J., Ganellin, C. R. and Parsons, M. E. (1972) *Nature (London)* 236, 385–390
3 Rendic, S., Sunjic, V., Toso, R. and Kajfez, F. (1979) *Xenobiotica,* 9, 555–564
4 Arunlakshana, O. and Schild, H. O. (1959) *Br. J. Pharmac. Chemother.* 14, 48–58
5 Parson, M. E. (1969) in *Quantitative Studies of Drug-Induced Gastric Secretion*, Ph.D. Thesis, University of London
6 Daly, M. J., Humphray, J. M. and Stables, R. (1980) *Gut,* 21, 408–412
7 Daly, M. J., Humphray, J. M. and Stables, R. (1979) *Gut,* 20, A914
8 Brittain, R. T., Daly, M. J. and Sutherland, M. (1980) *J. Pharm. Pharmacol.* 32, 76P
9 Bell, J. A., Gower, A. J., Martin, L. E., Mills, C. E. N. and Smith, W. P. (1981) *Biochem. Soc. Trans.* 9, 113
10 Shapira, M., Hagie, L., Cohen, I., Maxwell, V. and Isenberg, J. I. (1980) *Clin. Res.* 28, 72A
11 Comisso, G., Toso, R., Gratton, G., Kajfez, F. and Sunjic, V. (1979) *Acta Pharm. Jugoslav.* 29, 125–130
12 Meyers, W. M. and Peterson, W. L. (1980) *Clin. Res.* 28, 30A
13 Mills, J. G., Melvin, D. A., Griffiths, R., Hunt, H., Burland, W. L. and Milton-Thompson, G. J. (1980) *Gut,* 21, A462

Direct binding studies of adenosine receptors

Ulrich Schwabe

Institut für Pharmakologie und Toxikologie der Universität Bonn, Reuterstraße 2 b, 5300 Bonn 1, F.R.G.

Adenosine research has attracted increasing interest in the last decade for several reasons. Endogenous adenosine was discovered as a modulator of adenylate cyclase activity, as a possible neurotransmitter in the CNS and in peripheral smooth muscle tissue and as an important link in defects of purine metabolism associated with certain immunodeficiency diseases. Metabolically-stable adenosine analogues have been developed which facilitate the investigation of physiological and pharmacological effects of adenosine.

A first biochemical basis for the study of the molecular mechanism of adenosine action was discovered in 1970, when Sattin and Rall[1] observed that exogenous adenosine and some adenine nucleotides were potent stimulators of cyclic AMP accumulation in brain slices. These authors proposed the existence of an external adenosine receptor which stimulates adenylate cyclase in a hormone-like manner and is competitively inhibited by several methylxanthines.

2 years later the concept of purinergic nerves was developed by Burnstock[2] from the effects of adenine nucleotides and adenosine on peripheral tissues. Evidence supporting the hypothesis included observations that adenosine triphosphate was synthesized, stored and released from nonadrenergic noncholinergic nerves supplying several smooth muscle tissues and that it mimicked the effects of nerve stimulation on these tissues. Later Burnstock[3] suggested that it was possible to distinguish two types of purinergic receptors on the basis of four criteria: relative potencies of agonists and of competitive antagonists, changes in cyclic AMP levels and induction of prostaglandin synthesis. According to this classification P_1 purinergic receptors are most sensitive to adenosine and less sensitive to ATP, are blocked by methylxanthines and are linked to the adenylate cyclase. P_2 purinergic receptors are most sensitive to ATP, less sensitive to adenosine and are blocked by quinidine, 2-substituted imidazolines, 2'2'-pyridylisatogen and possibly apamin. The occupation is assumed to induce a stimulation of prostaglandin synthesis. However, more recent evidence shows that the antagonists of the P_2 receptors act noncompetitively and have undesirable nonspecific effects. Furthermore, no concrete concept has been proposed for the mechanisms by which a stimulation of P_2 purinergic receptors would be translated into physiological responses.

The effects of adenosine on the cyclic AMP system have been studied in a great variety of tissues and several subclasses of adenosine receptors have been identified by the use of adenosine analogues which differ functionally and pharmacologically. In the last year the first direct identification of adenosine receptors with radioligands was successfully performed in several laboratories. Several radioligands have been used and it is the aim of this article to give a first summary of the data obtained by this method. Before discussing the labeling of adenosine receptors by various radioligands it is necessary briefly to review the development which led to the classification of adenosine receptor subtypes.

Classification of adenosine receptor subtypes

Since the first description of a cyclic AMP increase elicited by adenosine in brain, several other tissues have been shown to respond similarly to adenosine. Sensitive responses were observed in human platelets, neuroblastoma cells, human astrocytoma cells, Leydig tumor cells, lymphocytes, bone cells, adrenal cells and turkey erythrocytes with half maximal activating concentrations ranging from 1 to 10 μM adenosine. In other cells adenosine was found to inhibit cyclic AMP accumulation, exceptionally low concentrations (5 nM) being effective in isolated fat cells. Contradictory results were reported from studies with ventricular myocardium which showed both an increase and decrease of cyclic AMP concentration in the presence of adenosine.

From studies with inhibitors of adenosine uptake like dipyridamole and p-nitrobenzylthioguanosine, which in intact cellular systems increase the effects of adenosine on cyclic AMP levels rather than reduce it, it was concluded that adenosine acts on an external plasma membrane receptor. Similarly, evidence for an adenosine site on the external cell surface has been obtained from studies with large molecular weight adenosine derivatives in coronary arteries.

In cell membrane preparations a direct stimulation or inhibition of adenylate cyclase activity by adenosine has been demonstrated (Table I). In many cases biphasic stimulatory and inhibitory effects of the nucleoside have been reported in the same membrane preparation. The first example of this observation was a particulate fraction from human platelets in which low concentrations of adenosine (2–25 μM) stimulated adenylate cyclase activity while higher concentrations (>100 μM) inhibited the enzyme[4]. As further shown in Table I virtually all adenylate cyclase preparations which have been examined are inhibited by adenosine, although the inhibition occurred only at relatively high concentrations of the nucleoside (0.1–1 mM). Both actions of adenosine were interpreted as independent processes mediated by different components of a receptor adenylate cyclase complex. Activation might possibly be produced via an external receptor and inhibition via the catalytic moiety of the adenylate cyclase.

This initial concept of two distinct adenosine reactive sites has been confirmed by the use of several adenosine agonists and antagonists in various tissue preparations. Many physiological responses of adenosine on blood pressure, coronary

TABLE I. Stimulation and inhibition of adenylate cyclase by adenosine in various tissues

Tissue	Stimulation EC$_{50}$ (μM)	Inhibition IC$_{50}$ (μM)
Pig coronary smooth muscle	0.01	>100
Rat striatum	0.5	50–100
Mouse neuroblastoma cells	1	>50
Turkey erythrocytes	1	
Human platelets	1–2	>500
Cultured human cells	3–5	>300
Leydig tumor cells	5–7	
Rat fetal bone cells	5–10	>100
Mouse thymocytes	10	
Rat mast cells	10	
Beef kidney medulla	20	
Adrenal tumor cells	25	
Rat fat cells		0.01
Cultured mouse brain cells		0.05
Rat liver		24–1000
Guinea pig lung		200–1000
Ehrlich tumor cells		1000
Rabbit small intestine		1000

EC$_{50}$: concentration at half maximal stimulation, IC$_{50}$: concentration at 50% inhibition.

blood flow, heart rate and renal blood flow are well known to be competitively antagonized by methylxanthines. The antagonism of adenosine actions by methylxanthines has also been demonstrated on cyclic AMP formation in intact cells as well as on adenylate cyclase activity in cell membrane preparations. In all systems which are stimulated by adenosine, theophylline inhibited adenylate cyclase. The adenosine antagonism occurred at 10–100 fold lower concentrations of theophylline than those which inhibit phosphodiesterase activity. Therefore, it has been concluded that the therapeutically important effects of the methylxanthines which are commonly ascribed to an inhibition of cyclic AMP breakdown, may in fact be due to an antagonism of theophylline against the stimulatory effects of endogenous adenosine on adenylate cyclase[5]. The inhibitory effects of high concentrations of adenosine on adenylate cyclase were not antagonized by theophylline.

The second approach to delineate the adenosine receptor subtypes was to use the relative potency of a variety of adenosine derivatives. Londos and Wolff[6] classified the adenosine receptors into P-site and R-site receptors. This classification was based on the characteristic pharmacological profile of two groups of adenosine derivatives which displayed opposing effects on the adenylate cyclase activity of Leydig tumor cells and of rat liver. Compounds with an intact ribose moiety of the adenosine molecule and modifications of the purine ring, such as 2-methyladenosine, 2-amino adenosine, N^6-methyladenosine and N^6-phenylisopropyladenosine (PIA), stimulated the Leydig cell cyclase but not the rat liver cyclase. Compounds with an intact purine moiety and modifications of the ribose ring, such as 2'-deoxyadenosine, 2',5'-dideoxyadenosine, 9-β-D-arabinofuranosyl adenine and 9-β-D-xylofuranosyl adenine, inhibited the liver cell cyclase and had only marginal effects on the Leydig tumor cell cyclase. Thus, compounds with an intact ribose ring were assumed to act on a 'ribose site' (R site) at the external cell surface and compounds with an intact purine ring were thought to act on a 'purine site' (P site) at the internal cell wall. The available information suggests that the R site mediates the physiologically and pharmacologically important actions of low extracellular concentrations of adenosine on intact cells. This process is antagonized by theophylline. The great majority of responses to adenosine and R-type analogues of adenosine are stimulatory on cyclic AMP formation via a GTP-dependent process, but in some cell types adenosine acts at the cell surface on an R site receptor to inhibit the activation of adenylate cyclase by hormones. Again, this inhibitory R site mediated process is GTP-dependent and antagonized by methylxanthines.

The P site receptor for adenosine of the adenylate cyclase is located at the internal surface of the cell membrane, probably associated with a regulatory unit of the catalytic component which remains intact on solubilization of membranes with neutral detergents. The effects of adenosine and P-type analogues of adenosine on this site are solely inhibitory and have been found in all tissues so far examined. Methylxanthines do not antagonize the P site effects. At present, physiological actions of adenosine cannot be attributed to the P site receptor.

The R site receptors for adenosine that mediate activation and inhibition of adenylate cyclase have further been discriminated with selected adenosine analogues. 5'-N-Ethylcarboxyamideadenosine (NECA) is a more potent agonist for stimulatory effects of adenosine on adenylate cyclase activity than is PIA, whereas the reverse order of potency is seen with the inhibitory responses to adenosine[7]. The potency of adenosine and 2-chloroadenosine was found to be intermediate between the potencies of these two analogues. Based on these observations the previous nomenclature of adenosine receptors has been extended by two new subclasses. The stimulatory R site adenosine receptor was termed R_a and the inhibitory receptor R_i[7]. In an earlier communication which described inhibitory effects of adenosine in cultured mouse brain cells another nomenclature was proposed, using the term A1-receptor for the one that mediates the inhibition and A2 for the one that mediates the stimulation of cyclic AMP accumulation[8].

Development of radioligands for adenosine receptors

For the characterization of these distinct types of adenosine receptors the measurement of physiological or biochemical responses of relative potencies of agonists and antagonists have been utilized. An alternative method of estimating receptor affinities for adenosine and related compounds is to measure their competition for receptor binding of radiolabeled compounds. The first attempts to identify adenosine receptors directly by radioligand binding studies were performed with radioactively-labeled adenosine. Reports have described experiments utilizing membrane preparations from rat fat cells[9], dog heart muscle[10], rat brain[11] and coronary and carotid arteries[12]. Although some binding characteristics were obtained, the adenosine sites differed considerably from the properties expected of adenosine receptors on the basis of the biological activities of adenosine and its analogues. Low binding affinities with dissociation constants ranging from 0.6 to 14 μM, unusually large numbers of binding sites and low specific binding indicated the failure to label physiologically relevant adenosine receptors. The main difficulties emerged from the extensive metabolism of [^{3}H]adenosine, the impossibility of discriminating between R site and P site adenosine receptors and the existence of a large number of nonreceptor binding sites. Unsatisfactory results were also obtained with [^{3}H]adenosinecyclopropylcarboxamide[13] and [^{3}H]-5'-adenylimidodiphosphate[14].

From these results it has been concluded that it is necessary to use radiolabeled adenosine analogues which are resistant to adenosine deaminase and other adenosine metabolizing enzymes and which are selective for R site or P site receptors. In the last year a variety of radiolabeled purine compounds has been used sucessfully for binding studies of adenosine receptors[15-19]. Among these radioligands 2-chloro[^{3}H]adenosine, (−)N^6-[^{3}H]phenylisopropyladenosine ([^{3}H]PIA) and N^6-[^{3}H]cyclohexyladenosine ([^{3}H]CHA) are adenoside agonists, the xanthine derivative 1,3-diethyl-8-[^{3}H]phenylxanthine ([^{3}H]DPX) is an adenosine antagonist.

All these compounds fulfil the first important prerequisite of metabolic stability against adenosine deaminase. This property appears to be important for two reasons. The first one has already been mentioned and refers to the possible degradation of the radioligands by endogenous enzymes. The second reason refers to the possible influence of endogenous adenosine on ligand binding to adenosine receptors and the necessity to pretreat the membrane preparations with exogenous adenosine deaminase. In adenosine deaminase-treated membranes specific binding of all new radioligands was two to four fold higher than in untreated membranes whereas nonspecific binding was not changed[16-19]. Furthermore, the adenosine deaminase treatment increases binding specificity, since in untreated rat brain membranes 2-chloro[^{3}H]adenosine binding was displaced by inosine, hypoxanthine and adenine[15]. All these compounds are devoid of adenosine-like activity in adenylate cyclase preparations or other adenosine sensitive systems. The effect of adenosine deaminase treatment is probably due to removal of endogenous adenosine still present in the repeatedly washed membrane preparations. However, the presence of adenosine deaminase creates additional problems in the interpretation of the results. The adenosine deaminase resistant analogues may behave as competitive inhibitors of the enzyme and thus increase the amount of endogenous adenosine. But many compounds which displace binding are neither substrates nor inhibitors of adenosine deaminase. The other possibility is that the radioligands may bind to the enzyme attached to the membranes and would mimic an increased amount of receptor binding. Both possibilities have been carefully checked by the variation of membrane concentrations and by the use of the adenosine deaminase inhibitor deoxycoformycin[16,19]. The available evidence suggests that the radioligands do not bind to the added adenosine deaminase. Thus, under the experimental condition of the radioligand binding assay approximately 50–70% of the adenosine receptors appear to be occupied by small amounts of endogenous adenosine which cannot be removed by washing of the membranes. This condition may be an additional important reason for the failure to label physiologically relevant adenosine receptors with [^{3}H]adenosine.

Another consideration concerning the level of occupancy of adenosine receptors should briefly be discussed. Probably, most of the endogenous adenosine may be generated and attached to the binding sites during the preparation procedure of the cell membranes. However, it is not unlikely that a high degree of receptor occupancy by the endogenous nucleoside reflects a condition which may also occur in intact cells under physiological conditions. An interesting example is provided by isolated fat cells, in which nanomolar amounts of adenosine are released in the basal state and a marked lipolytic response is elicited upon addition of adenosine deaminase[20]. Preliminary results indicate that *in vivo*, radioligand binding is increased following a pretreatment with adenosine deaminase.

The binding data obtained with four different radioligands in several tissues are listed in Table II. The binding of each of these ligands to sites in membranes is rapid, reversible, saturable and stereospecific as demonstrated by the stereoisomers of PIA. The binding of all radioligands displays the specificity and affinity of binding to true adenosine receptors.

Both the dissociation constants and the maximal number of binding sites are several orders of magnitude lower than the corresponding values previously reported

TABLE II. Radioligands used for identification of adenosine receptors

Radioligand	Tissue	K_D nM	B_{max} fmol mg^{-1} protein	Reference
2-Chloro[^{3}H]adenosine	Rat brain	23.5	476	15
		1.3	207	18
		16	380	18
N^6-Cyclohexyl[^{3}H]adenosine	Guinea pig brain	6	370*	16
	Bovine brain	0.3	340*	16
		1.8	200*	16
(−)N^6-[^{3}H]Phenylisopropyladenosine	Rat brain	5	810	17
	Rat fat cells	6	1900	19
1,3-Diethyl-8-[^{3}H]phenylxanthine	Guinea pig brain	70	500*	16
	Bovine brain	5	1000*	16

* B_{max} values recalculated on the basis 1 g brain tissue equivalent to 100 mg protein.

for [³H]adenosine binding. The density of 200–2000 fmol mg⁻¹ of adenosine receptor binding sites is comparable to that of several other hormones and neurotransmitters. The relatively high B_{max} values for [³H]PIA binding in brain and fat cell membranes were measured at higher temperatures (37°C) than those for the binding of the other radioligands (23–25°C) and, therefore, are probably due to the distinct temperature dependence of [³H]PIA binding and not to the labeling of a different population of adenosine receptors.

The dissociation constants are in the range of 0.3–70 nM for all radioligands. Although the experimental conditions are not fully comparable for these data, the relatively broad concentration range is suggestive of a heterogenous mixture of two or more different types of adenosine receptor sites. In fact, two binding sites have been described for 2-chloro-[³H]adenosine in rat brain[18] and for [³H]CHA in bovine brain membranes[16]. Whether the high and low affinity sites may be attributed to different subclasses of adenosine receptors, has not yet been adequately explored. However, a first basic interpretation of the binding characteristics obtained with the four radioligands is possible. They all appear to label R site adenosine receptors, since the binding of the ligands is displaced by methylxanthines and typical R site agonists, both of which are inactive at P site receptors. Furthermore, P site agonists, such as 2′,5′-dideoxyadenosine do not substantially inhibit the binding of the radioligands.

A further approach to delineate adenosine receptor subtypes by radioligand binding is to determine the proportion of R_a and R_i adenosine receptors by analysis of competition curves with subtype selective adenosine analogues. PIA has been classified as subtype selective for R_i receptors and NECA as selective for R_a receptors[7]. All hitherto performed binding studies have shown that PIA most effectively displaced radioligand binding with the only exception of guinea-pig brain membranes in which 2-chloroadenosine was the most potent displacer of [³H]DPX binding. NECA was 40 fold less potent than PIA as an inhibitor of 2-chloro[³H]adenosine binding[18]. From these results it may be concluded that the two N⁶-substituted adenosine analogues and 2-chloroadenosine appear to label R_i adenosine receptors. As to be expected [³H]PIA appears to be very good, and at the present the most useful, radioligand for studying R_i receptors. The importance of [³H]PIA as a selective ligand for R_i receptors is further suggested by the results obtained with rat fat cell membranes. This cell type is considered R_i selective on the basis of physiological data and has a high affinity for [³H]PIA[19]. Thus, fat cell membranes offer the advantage of enabling study of radioligand binding to R_i receptors without interference by R_a receptors, whereas in membrane preparations from whole brain, both receptor subtypes may contribute to overall radioligand binding[8]. From the data available at present it cannot finally be estimated whether [³H]PIA is a completely subtype selective radioligand for R_i receptors since R_a selective tissues have so far not been studied.

[³H]DPX is an antagonist ligand and at present the only radioligand which, in one tissue at least, appears to label R_a adenosine receptor sites. The competition curves obtained with [³H]DPX in guinea pig brain membranes showed that the R_i agonist CHA displaced about 40% of the radioligand binding at nanomolar concentrations and the remaining 60% only at high micromolar concentrations of the CHA[16]. This may indicate that 40% of specific binding is to R_i receptors and the remaining 60% is to R_a receptors. In agreement with this interpretation, the nonselective R site agonist 2-chloroadenosine was 75 fold more potent than PIA in displacing [³H]DPX binding and the stereoisomers of

PIA showed no stereoselective inhibition of the radioligand binding[16].

Adenosine sensitive adenylate cyclase systems are characterized by the fact that guanine nucleotides such as GTP or its nonhydrolysable analogue GMPP(NH)P are required for stimulation as well as for inhibition of the enzyme[7]. It is also known that binding of ligands to hormone receptors associated with adenylate cyclase is frequently regulated by guanine nucleotides which selectively decrease affinities of agonists but not of antagonists. A similar observation has been reported for the binding of the adenosine analogue [^{3}H]CHA to brain membranes. The specific binding of [^{3}H]CHA was displaced by submicromolar concentrations of the guanine nucleotides[16]. This pattern of guanine nucleotide effects suggests a strong analogy with the mechanisms at most neurotransmitter and hormone receptors linked to adenylate cyclase.

Possible future developments

The data reviewed here show that the efforts to identify and characterize adenosine receptors by direct ligand binding techniques are just at their beginning. Up to now, binding data have been presented for brain and fat cell membranes. Both tissues provided a reasonable model to study the properties of adenosine receptors, since the biochemical effects of adenosine and its analogues on adenylate cyclase had been sufficiently characterized. Several other tissues, in which subtypes of adenosine receptors have been defined on the basis of adenylate cyclase studies, will be the next promising candidates for further binding studies. Particular interest will focus on the possibility of defining cellular systems which contain only one of the adenosine receptor subtypes. To date, only rat fat cells have been shown to contain exclusively R_i receptors whereas R_a subtype selective cells have not yet been described. However, it is suggested by a great deal of data, that platelets, lymphocytes and mast cells predominantly contain R_a receptors. Therefore, the use of these cells in binding studies will facilitate the search for R_a subtype selective radioligands.

Another approach for discriminating between adenosine receptor subtypes more accurately would be to develop adenosine antagonists which were either R_a or R_i selective. At present, methylxanthines are the only R site antagonists available. Compounds such as isobutylmethylxanthine, theophylline, and caffeine which distinguish between P site and R site adenosine receptors, are not selective for R_a and R_i receptor subtypes. In analogy with other receptor systems subtype selective antagonists would provide an important tool for the study of adenosine receptors.

The concept of subclasses of adenosine receptors and the development of subtype selective antagonists could have interesting implications for drug therapy. As an important example, theophylline can be mentioned as one of the mainstays of therapy in acute bronchospasm and obstructive pulmonary diseases. Although inhibition of phosphodiesterase and alterations in intracellular calcium metabolism have long been considered as the basis of the therapeutic action of the methylxanthines, recent evidence demonstrates that an antagonistic interaction with adenosine receptors may contribute to the beneficial effects of theophylline[5]. At present, it is not known which subtype of adenosine receptors may be involved in the broncholytic action of theophylline, but subtype selective antagonists could result in therapeutic advances of the type encountered in the pursuit of selective agonists and antagonists for other hormone and drug receptors.

In conclusion, the first direct binding studies have provided a new approach to investigating adenosine receptors. It will be interesting to see whether an extension of these studies to other cellular systems and the development of further subtype selective radioligands will yield greater insights into the physiological and molecular properties of adenosine receptors.

Reading list

1 Sattin, A. and Rall, T. W. (1970) *Mol. Pharmacol.* 6, 13–23
2 Burnstock, G. (1972) *Pharmacol. Rev.* 24, 509–581
3 Burnstock, G. (1979) in *Physiological and Regulatory Functions of Adenosine and Adenine Nucleotides* (Baer, H. P. and Drummond, G. I., eds), pp. 3–32
4 Haslam, R. J. and Lynham, J. A. (1972) *Life Sci.* 11, 1143–1154
5 Fredholm, B. B. (1980) *Trends Pharmacol. Sci.* 2, 129–132
6 Londos, C. and Wolff, J. (1977) *Proc. Natl Acad. Sci. U.S.A.* 74, 5482–5486
7 Londos, C., Cooper, D. M. F. and Wolff, J. (1980) *Proc. Natl Acad. Sci. U.S.A.* 77, 2551–2554
8 Van Calker, D., Müller, M. and Hamprecht, B. (1978) *Nature (London)* 276, 839–841
9 Malbon, C. C., Hert, R. C. and Fain, J. N. (1978) *J. Biol. Chem.* 253, 3114–3122
10 Dutta, P. and Mustafa, S. J. (1979) *J. Pharmacol. Exp. Ther.* 211, 496–501
11 Schwabe, U., Kiffe, H., Puchstein, C. and Trost, T. (1979) *Naunyn-Schmiedebergs Arch. Pharmakol.* 310, 59–67
12 Dutta, P. and Mustafa, S. J. (1980) *J. Pharmacol. Exp. Ther.* 214, 496–502
13 Daly, J. W., Nimitkitpaisan, Y., Pons, F., Bruns, R. F. Smellie, F. and Skolnick, P. (1979) *Pharmacologist* 21, 253
14 Williams, M. and Risley, E. A. (1980) *Fed. Proc. Fed. Am. Soc. Exp. Biol.* 39, 1009
15 Wu, P. H., Phillis, J. W., Balls, K. and Rinaldi, B. (1980) *Can. J. Physiol. Pharmacol.* 58, 576–579
16 Bruns, R. F., Daly, J. W. and Snyder, S. H. (1980) *Proc. Natl Acad. Sci. U.S.A.* 77, 5547–5551
17 Schwabe, U. and Trost, T. (1980) *Naunyn-Schmiedebergs Arch. Pharmakol.* 313, 179–187
18 Williams, M. and Risley, E. A. (1980) *Proc. Natl Acad. Sci. U.S.A.* 77, 6892–6896
19 Trost, T. and Schwabe, U. (1981) *Mol Pharmacol.* 19, 228–235
20 Schwabe, U., Ebert, R. and Erbler, H. C. (1975) in *Advances in Cyclic Nucleotide Research* (Drummond, G. I., Greengard, P. and Robison, G. A., eds), Vol. 5, pp. 569–584, Raven Press, New York

The controversial problem of insulin action

Otto Walaas and Robert S. Horn

Institute of Medical Biochemistry, University of Oslo, Norway

It is well established that insulin exerts numerous effects on the metabolism of carbohydrates, lipids and amino acids as well as on membrane transport processes. However, in spite of extensive studies the mechanism of insulin action at the molecular level is an unsolved problem[1]. At the present time there is general agreement that the initial event in insulin action involves binding of the hormone to specific membrane receptors in target cells. A milestone in this field was the identification of the insulin receptor in the early 1970s[2,3]. The binding of insulin to its receptor initiates rapid changes in membrane transport and changes of the activity of intracellular enzymes as well as long term effects on protein synthesis. However, the coupling system between insulin and the effector system is still largely unknown. A series of small molecules have been proposed as 'second messenger' such as cyclic AMP, cyclic GMP, Ca^{2+}, hydrogen peroxide as well as unknown nucleotides. Until now these investigations have been rather unsuccessful. Numerous investigations have failed to demonstrate any correlation between the effect of insulin on the level of cyclic AMP or cyclic GMP and the metabolic effects of insulin under the same conditions. Release of Ca^{2+} may be of importance to the insulin effect on membrane transport as proposed by Clausen. However, there is no indication that Ca^{2+} release is a primary mediator in insulin action on intracellular systems. During the last few years some progress has been made in this field by investigations along two different lines.

The action of insulin on reversible phosphorylation of enzymes and other proteins

Many acute effects of insulin upon metabolism involve pathways regulated by protein kinases and protein phosphatases. Control of reversible enzyme phosphorylation by insulin was first discovered by Larner and co-workers in the early 1960s. It was demonstrated that insulin in muscle increased the activity of glycogen synthase when measured in the absence of G-6-P, and that this effect could be attributed to a dephosphorylation of the enzyme. Today, it is strongly indicated that regulation of phosphorylation–dephosphorylation of enzymes represents an important mechanism in the control of enzyme activities by insulin. Insulin has been shown to promote dephosphorylation of several metabolic enzymes such as glycogen synthase, pyruvate dehydrogenase, hydroxymethylglutaryl CoA reductase and reductase kinase[4]. The most extensive investigation relevant to this problem has been done on the glycogen synthase and pyruvate dehydrogenase systems.

The glycogen synthase system

During the last few years it has been

shown by Cohen[4] and associates that phosphorylation–dephosphorylation of this enzyme is subjected to complex regulation by kinases and phosphatases. The enzyme is phosphorylated by three different kinases and dephosphorylated by several protein phosphatases, the most important being protein phosphatase-1. The latter enzyme is inhibited by heat stable inhibitor proteins, and the inhibitory activity of inhibitor-1 is dependent upon phosphorylation by cyclic AMP-dependent protein kinase. The intriguing question is how insulin can promote dephosphorylation of synthase by influencing this complex regulatory system. In the early 1970s it was shown by Larner and co-workers[5] as well as in our own[6] laboratory that insulin treatment of diaphragm resulted in decreased activity of the cyclic AMP-dependent protein kinase. It has also been shown that insulin exerts similar effects in adipose tissue. Recent work by Cohen and collaborators[4] has brought inhibitor-1 into focus for insulin action. It was demonstrated that insulin *in vivo* decreases the phosphorylation of inhibitor-1. This would lead to increased activity of protein phosphatase-1 with increased synthase activity. The problem has been further complicated by the newly discovered protein phosphatase[4] which is activated by ATP-Mg in the presence of a protein factor; apparently a kinase. It remains to be seen if this phosphatase is activated by insulin as suggested by Cohen[4]. At present it seems that the insulin mediated dephosphorylation of glycogen synthase may be promoted by a double effect, both inhibition of cyclic AMP-dependent protein kinase and activation of protein phosphatase.

The pyruvate dehydrogenase system

Pyruvate dehydrogenase is inactivated by phosphorylation and activated by dephosphorylation of the catalytic subunit of $M_r = 42,000$. In adipose tissue lipolytic hormones enhance phosphorylation while insulin promotes dephosphorylation of the enzyme. Recently, the mechanism of this action of insulin has been studied by Jarett[7] and co-workers in a subcellular mixture of plasma membranes and mitochondria isolated from adipocytes. Direct addition of insulin to this mixture resulted in decreased phosphorylation and increased activity of the enzyme, and it was shown that this action of insulin was due to stimulation of pyruvate dehydrogenase phosphatase. It has been proposed that insulin activates the enzyme by release of Ca^{2+} in the mitochondria, but this has not been proven.

The effect of insulin on phosphorylation of other proteins

Avruch and co-workers demonstrated that insulin stimulates ^{32}P-incorporation from ^{32}P-γ-ATP into a cytosol protein $M_r = 123,000$ in adipocytes and hepatocytes, and this protein has been identified as ATP–citrate lyase. A dramatic effect of insulin has been demonstrated on the pre-adipocyte cell line 3T3–L1[8]. During differentiation these cells acquire a high concentration of insulin receptors and an insulin-sensitive hexose uptake system. Insulin promotes a 20-fold increase in the phosphorylation of the ribosomal protein S6 of $M_r = 31,000$. This effect could also be demonstrated in cell-free extracts from insulin-treated cells. Recent investigations have demonstrated that insulin influences the phosphorylation of a large series of proteins in different compartments of the cell. Some of these insulin effects can be explained as antagonistic against phosphorylations promoted by cyclic AMP-dependent protein kinases. However, insulin also promotes increased as well as decreased phosphorylation of proteins by mechanisms which are not yet identified.

Recently proposed mechanisms of insulin action

In spite of extensive efforts investigations have failed to identify the coupling system between the insulin-receptor complex and the influence of the hormone on enzymes and membranes. However, some progress has been made during the last few years mainly by investigations along three different lines.

Internalization of the insulin–receptor complex

It has been demonstrated that insulin, after binding to membrane receptors, is rapidly internalized by a process of receptor mediated endocytosis[9]. The internalized insulin mainly associates with lysosomes, and internalization of insulin with its receptor may underlie the phenomenon of 'down regulation'. It appears that the receptor mediated degradation of insulin discovered by Terris and Steiner now can be attributed to its processing by lysosomes. The hypothesis that the degraded fragments of insulin can act as a 'second messenger' has, however, received little support until now. Lysosomotropic drugs which block degradation of internalized insulin have no inhibitory effect on the metabolic actions of the hormone. Further evidence against this hypothesis are the findings that compounds such as Concanavalin A, antibodies against insulin receptor and hydrogen peroxide trigger a large series of metabolic effects which closely resemble those of insulin. It should be pointed out that during the internalization, whole fragments of the plasma membrane are processed intracellularly. Some intracellular insulin effects may perhaps be expressed by these membrane fragments. Suzuki and Kono[10] recently made the interesting observation that a fraction of glucose transport activity is associated with the Golgi apparatus in adipocytes. Incubation of cells with insulin led to translocation of the intracellular transport activity to the plasma membrane. This process may be part of the mechanism by which insulin stimulates cellular glucose transport.

Phosphorylation of membrane proteins

It has been shown that insulin influences membrane protein phosphorylation in muscle, liver and adipose tissue. We have recently reported that direct addition of insulin to isolated sarcolemma membranes from skeletal muscle increases phosphorylation of a membrane protein $M_r = 16,000$. This effect was attributed to activation of a cyclic AMP-independent protein kinase. Furthermore, the insulin effect was enhanced 3-fold in the presence of μM GTP[11]. It is indicated that GTP, probably through a GTP-binding protein, acts as a modulator in the action of insulin on this sarcolemma membrane protein kinase. The phosphorylated membrane protein $M_r = 16,000$ is soluble in acid chloroform/methanol and has been identified as a proteolipid. The amino acid composition is characterized by a high degree of hydrophobic residues, and is rather similar to the amino acid composition of proteolipids isolated from purified $(Na^+ + K^+)$-ATPases. Racker has proposed that proteolipids function as ionophores in membranes by forming channels for the transport of protons and ions. Green[12] and coworkers recently demonstrated that phospholipids can act as ionophores for ions, sugars and amino acids and proposed that phospholipids bound to proteins act as the physiological ionophores for solute molecules. The phosphorylated proteolipid $M_r = 16,000$ may, therefore, be part of an effector system for membrane transport. Increased phosphorylation of the proteolipid promoted by insulin may increase the activity of the transport system. Similarly, it has been shown that increased transport activity in erythrocytes is correlated with increased phosphorylation of a specific protein.

Towards identification of the 'second messenger'?

Over the years many unsuccessful attempts have been made to identify the

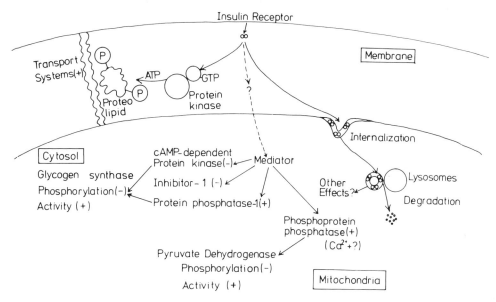

Fig. 1. The model illustrates a proposed mechanism for the action of insulin. The insulin—receptor complex triggers release of a mediator which regulates phosphorylation of enzymes by control of protein phosphatase and protein kinase activities. A second effector system for the insulin—receptor complex is activation of a membrane protein kinase with GTP as a modulator. The subsequent increased phosphorylation of a membrane proteolipid is causally linked to the increase of transport processes. Internalization of the insulin—receptor complex may not be involved in insulin action but terminates the hormonal effect. Some of the statements are hypothetical. (+) and (−) designate increased and decreased activity of phosphorylation.

unknown 'second messenger' of insulin action. It is, therefore, of the greatest interest that Larner[13] and co-workers recently isolated from skeletal muscle a material which could mimic the action of insulin on some intracellular enzymes. The material was extracted from rabbit and rat skeletal muscle and tentatively identified as a small molecular peptide Mr = 1000–1500. It was shown that this material inhibited cyclic AMP-dependent protein kinase and activated glycogen synthase phosphatase. Increased activity of the same fraction was obtained by pretreatment of the muscle with insulin. Jarett[14,15] and co-workers have isolated a similar material from adipocytes and adipocyte plasma membranes. This material mimicked the action of insulin on the pyruvate dehydrogenase system. Furthermore, the activity of the isolated fraction was increased by pretreatment of the adipocytes with insulin. It was demonstrated that insulin increased the activity of pyruvate dehydrogenase in a subcellular system composed of plasma membrane and mitochondria, but had no effect on mitochondria in the absence of membranes. The isolated peptide material could substitute for insulin + plasma membranes and stimulate pyruvate dehydrogenase by direct interaction with mitochondria. The work by Larner and Jarett represents a new promising approach in this field.

Future trends and unsolved problems

A proposed model of insulin action is shown in Fig. 1. There is general agreement that an important mechanism in the action of insulin on intracellular enzymes involves control of protein phosphorylation. Dephosphorylation and subsequent activation of these enzymes due to insulin have been attributed to increase of protein phosphatase as well as to inhibition of protein kinase activity. Opinions in this field are controversial, and future studies are needed in order to establish the detailed mechanism. The dogma that the action of insulin on intracellular enzymes is due to a mediator triggered by insulin–receptor interaction and released from the membrane is still widely accepted. The most promising candidate for this function is the peptide material recently isolated by Larner and Jarett. If this substance in future studies satisfies the criteria required for a hormonal messenger a major breakthrough in this field would have been accomplished. The observation that insulin directly stimulates membrane protein kinase with subsequent increased phosphorylation of a membrane proteolipid may be correlated with insulin stimulation of membrane transport processes. It remains to be shown that the increased membrane protein phosphorylation is causally involved in increased transport processes without participation of a small molecular mediator.

Reading list

1 Walaas, O. and Walaas, E. (1974) *Acta Endocrinol. (Copenhagen)* 77, Suppl. 191, 93–127
2 Roth, J. (1973) *Metabolism* 22, 1059–1073
3 Kahn, C. R. (1979) *Trends Biochem. Sci.* 4, N263–N266
4 Cohen, P. (1980) *Molecular Aspects of Cellular Regulation*, Vol. 1, North Holland, Amsterdam, London and New York
5 Shen, L. C., Villar-Palasi, C. and Larner, J. (1970) *Physiol. Chem. Phys.* 2, 536–544
6 Walaas, O., Walaas, E. and Grønnerød, O. (1973) *Eur. J. Biochem.* 40, 465–477
7 Seals, J. R., McDonald, J. M. and Jarett, L. (1979) *J. Biol. Chem.* 254, 6997–7001
8 Smith, C. J., Rubin, C. S. and Rosen, O. M. (1980) *Proc. Natl Acad. Sci. U.S.A.* 77, 2641–2645
9 Schlessinger, J. (1980) *Trends Biochem. Sci.* 5, 210–214
10 Suzuki, K. and Kono, T. (1980) *Proc. Natl Acad. Sci. U.S.A.* 77, 2542–2545
11 Walaas, O., Walaas, E., Lystad, E., Alertsen, Aa. R. and Horn, R. S. (1979) *Mol. Cell. Endocrinol.* 16, 45–55
15 Green, D. E., Fry, M. and Blondin, G. A. (1980) *Proc. Natl Acad. Sci. U.S.A.* 77, 257–261
13 Larner, J., Galasko, G., Cheng, K., DePaoli-Roach, A. A., Huang, L., Daggy, P. and Kellogg, J. (1979) *Science* 206, 1408–1410
14 Jarett, L. and Seals, J. R. (1979) *Science* 206, 1407–1408
15 Kiechle, F. L., Jarett, L., Popp, D. A. and Kotagal, N. (1980) *Diabetes* 29, 852–855

Addendum: Recent developments

Conflicting results on the effect of insulin on protein phosphorylation continue to appear. The work by Exton and co-workers is not consistent with the view that insulin increases protein phosphatase activity due to decreased phosphorylation of inhibitor-1 (Khatra. B. S., Chiasson, J.-L., Shikama, H., Exton, J. H. and Soderling, T. R. (1980) *FEBS Lett.* 114, 253–256). Furthermore, their work does not support the hypothesis that insulin activates glycogen synthase by producing an inhibitor of cyclic AMP-dependent protein kinase (Shikama, H., Chiasson, J.-L. and Exton, J. H. (1981) *J. Biol. Chem.* 256, 4450–4454). Further support for the hypothesis that insulin acts via membrane cyclic AMP-independent protein kinases has appeared. Direct addition of insulin to particulate preparations from 3T3-L1 adipocytes stimulated phosphorylation of S6 ribosomal protein (Rosen, D. M., Rubin, C. S., Cobb, M. H. and Smith, C. J. (1981) *J. Biol. Chem.* 256, 3630–3633). Denton and co-workers reported that cyclic AMP-independent protein kinase in adipocyte membranes phosphorylated acetyl CoA carboxylase at a site distinct from that phosphorylated by cyclic AMP-dependent protein kinase. The phosphorylation catalysed by cyclic AMP dependent protein kinase resulted in activation of the enzyme with characteristics identical to those seen after exposure of fat cells to insulin (Brownsey, R. W., Belsham, G. J. and Denton, R. M. (1981) *FEBS Lett.* 124, 145–150). In sarcolemma membranes, insulin stimulation of protein kinase activity was abolished by ADP-ribosylation of the membranes in the presence of cholera toxin and NAD^+ (Walaas, O., Horn, R. S. and Adler, A. (1981) *FEBS Lett.* 128, 133–136). Final resolution of problems concerned with insulin action on protein phosphorylation must await determination of specific site phosphorylation as well as purification of the enzymes concerned.

Release of peptide-like material from membranes due to insulin as discovered by Larner and by Jarett has been confirmed (Seals, J. R. and Czech, M. P. (1981) *J. Biol. Chem.* 256, 2894–2899). The material derived from adipocyte membranes stimulated pyruvate dehydrogenase and had an M_r of 2000–4000. Reports on the chemical structure of the material have not yet appeared. We recently reported that a phosphorylated subunit M_r 3600 containing 34 amino acids is derived from the insulin-dependent phosphorylated proteolipid M_r 15000 in sarcolemma membranes (Walaas, O., Sletten, K., Horn, R. S., Lystad, E., Adler, A. and Alertsen, Aa. R. (1981) *FEBS Lett.* 128, 137–141).

In adipocytes, insulin has been shown to increase the number of cytochalasin B binding sites in plasma membranes while the binding sites in the microsomal fraction were decreased, supporting the view that a translocation process may be involved in the action of insulin on sugar transport (Cushman, S. W. and Wardzala, L. J. (1980) *J. Biol. Chem.* 255, 4758–4762). Certainly, insulin action is still an unsolved problem.

The insulin receptor: structural features

Michael O. Czech, Joan Massague, Paul F. Pilch

Department of Biochemistry, University of Massachusetts Medical School, Worcester, MA 01605, U.S.A.
Department of Biochemistry, Boston University School of Medicine, Boston, MA 02118, U.S.A.

Recently developed affinity-labeling techniques have been used to study the subunit composition and stoichiometry of the insulin receptor. The minimum subunit structure deduced consists of two α and two β glycoprotein subunits, all disulfide-linked in a symmetrical receptor complex. This structure resembles the general design of immunoglobulin G molecules. When insulin binds to this complex the α subunit becomes more sensitive to exogenous protease, indicating that the conformation of the complex has been altered. Such structural information should help further define the molecular basis of insulin action.

Probably no hormone elicits as complex an array of physiological cellular responses in target tissues as insulin does. In the liver, muscle and adipose tissue, a number of enzymes involved in intermediary metabolism are regulated by insulin via both rapid modifications of proteins and the control of gene expression. All the rapidly responsive enzymes that have been well studied seem to be regulated in part by phosphorylation–dephosphorylation reactions. There is suggestive evidence that insulin action leads to the dephosphorylation of some cellular proteins and the phosphorylation of others. In addition, a number of transport systems for nutrients, such as hexoses and amino acids as well as certain ions, are modulated by this hormone. Again, these can be divided into modes of regulation that are either rapid or slow in onset. Several recent reviews are available that describe our current rather scanty understanding of the molecular basis of these actions of insulin[1-5].

A cell surface membrane component referred to as the insulin receptor is a key feature of our concept of how insulin acts. The receptor has a high affinity for insulin – it is generally agreed that the Ka is close to 1 nanomolar[6]. The number of high affinity receptors is quite low in all cell types. Even in tissues where it is most abundant, the insulin receptor represents only about 0.01% of the protein in plasma membrane preparations[7]. In spite of this relative paucity of insulin receptors on the cell surface, there appear to be many fold more than required to elicit maximal physiological responses in cells. Thus, binding of ^{125}I-insulin to about 5% or less of the high affinity receptor available on adipocytes causes maximal activation of glucose transport[8]. This phenomenon has been explained by the spare receptor hypothesis which suggests that all insulin receptors are equivalent but that the signal generated by only a small percentage is sufficient to elicit the physiological responses. However, there appear to be exceptions to this concept[9]. Variations in the number of receptor–ligand complexes required to elicit maximal biological responses could simply reflect different sensitivities of the responsive enzyme systems to the intracellular signals generated.

In addition to the responses involving enzymes and transporters several other cellular events are thought to be a consequence of insulin-receptor interaction. For example, a specific proteolytic degradation of the hormone appears to be mediated by a receptor-linked process[10]. Hormone binding to receptor also diminishes the number of receptors on cells[11] and the high concentrations of insulin in the circulation in certain physiological states such as obesity leads to a decrease in sensitivity of target tissues to the hormone[12,13]. This desensitization process is rather slow and probably reflects receptor-mediated endocytosis of the insulin–receptor complex[14]. An intriguing question is whether such internalized insulin receptors might be recycled back to the cell surface.

The ability of the receptor to bind insulin with high affinity has been conserved extremely well during evolution. Human insulin binds as well to receptors from the hagfish[15] (a species 500 million years old) as it does to the human receptor. Remarkably, hagfish insulin binds to hagfish receptor less well than does human insulin[15] indicating that the hormone molecule has experienced more extensive structural changes than has the receptor binding site.

Methodology for determining receptor structure

The binding characteristics for the insulin–receptor interaction have been exhaustively investigated, but until recently there was very little information about the structure of the receptor. Various new methods introduced by several groups have facilitated progress. Over 10 years ago Cuatrecasas initiated affinity-purification techniques involving immobilized insulin on agarose supports, but the amount of purified material obtained was exceedingly small[7]. Refinements to this approach allowed Jacobs et al.[16] to obtain receptor-rich fractions that exhibited a major protein band at about M_r 135,000 on sodium dodecyl sulfate polyacrylamide gels. However, the purity of these preparations was difficult to assess because binding activity was greatly diminished by the purification procedure.

Using new affinity-labeling techniques it has been possible to identify the insulin receptor and, in combination with affinity purification, to deduce its subunit composition and stoichiometry[17]. Yip and colleagues found that photo-activatable analogs of ^{125}I-insulin with azide groups at the B_1 and B_{29} positions could be used to affinity-label the receptor by flash photolysis[18–20]. Pilch and Czech affinity-labeled the insulin receptor using the cross-linking reagent disuccinimidyl suberate, which they synthesized[21,22]. ^{125}I-insulin was allowed to bind to intact cell or plasma membrane receptors and free hormone was washed from the insulin–receptor complexes at low temperature. When the cross-linking reagent was added, up to 30% of the bound ligand was covalently linked to receptor protein. The labeled receptor subunits were readily analysed by one- or two-dimensional sodium dodecyl sulfate polyacrylamide gel electrophoresis (SDS-

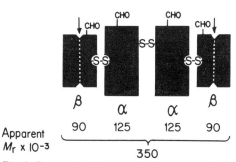

Fig. 1. Proposed minimum subunit structure for the insulin receptor. The key features of this recently deduced[17] structure are two copies of each of two glycoprotein subunit types, denoted α and β, disulfide bridges linking all subunits, and a high sensitivity of the β subunit to proteolytic cleavage near the center of the amino acid sequence (arrows). The presence of other subunits not covalently linked to this structure cannot as yet be excluded. The apparent molecular weight values refer to estimates obtained on SDS gels in the non-reduced (intact complex, M_r 350,000) and reduced state (individual subunits), respectively.

PAGE)[17,21-23]. More recently, antireceptor antibodies from patients with acanthosis nigricans and insulin resistance have been used for the specific immunoprecipitation of insulin receptors from detergent solution[24]. These antibodies compete with insulin for the insulin receptor. Initial attempts to purify the receptor with these reagents[24] immunoprecipitated peptides with lower molecular weights than those obtained by other methods[17,18,21], probably due to contaminating proteolytic activity. More recent work with these antibodies has confirmed the results obtained by affinity labeling[25].

General features of the insulin receptor structure

The minimum subunit composition of the receptor has been deduced from investigations in our laboratory using affinity-crosslinking[17,21-23,26,27] in combination with studies by Jacobs et al.[28-29] who used immobilized insulin for affinity purification (Fig. 1). The insulin receptor in all tissues studied is composed of at least four subunits that are disulfide-linked into a large receptor complex of apparent Mr 350,000[17,27]. Two of the subunits, referred to as α subunits[17], (Mr 125,000 on SDS-PAGE) are thought to be linked by one or more disulfide bridges. The two other subunits, denoted β[17], (Mr 90,000 upon gel electrophoresis) are disulfide linked to the α subunits (Fig. 1). The receptor complex exhibits a lower apparent molecular weight on SDS-PAGE than would be expected from its subunit composition; this is partly because intrachain disulfide bridges maintain a compact structure in detergent solution.

This subunit composition of $(\alpha\beta)_2$ is similar to that of immunoglobulin G molecules in that two heavy and two light chains are present in a symmetrical disulfide-linked structure. It is intriguing to note that immunoglobulins serve as immunogenic receptors on lymphocyte cell surfaces. Recently we have shown that a region near the middle of the β subunit is extremely sensitive to exogenous protease activity (Fig. 1, arrows)[17,27]. Since neuraminidase treatment alters the electrophoretic mobility of both subunits it appears that oligosaccharide chains containing sialic acid are attached to the α and β subunits[30]. This also suggests that both subunits are exposed on the exofacial surface of the cell membrane. Although the α subunit is normally more susceptible to affinity labeling than the β subunit, the exact location of specific insulin binding sites on this structure is not known. It seems reasonable to suggest that the insulin receptor complex is at least divalent, given the symmetry of the molecule, but this is not proven.

Classes of interchain disulfide bonds in the insulin receptor

The model in Fig. 1 shows at least two classes of interpeptide disulfide bonds in the $(\alpha\beta)_2$ receptor complex[17,26,31]. Class I comprises those disulfide bonds that link the two $(\alpha\beta)$ receptor fragments (or halves) and display a high susceptibility to reducing agents. Thus, when intact fat cells are successively treated with 1 mM dithiothreitol (DTT), ^{125}I-insulin, and a cross-linking agent such as disuccinimidyl suberate, all the affinity-labeled insulin receptors on the outer surface of these cells appear as $(\alpha\beta)$ fragments (Mr 210,000) upon SDS-PAGE. Fig. 2 illustrates the reaction whereby the $(\alpha\beta)_2$ receptor complex dissociates under these conditions (Reaction 1).

Class II disulfide bridges, namely those linking α and β subunits, are less sensitive to reduction. The dissociation of these bonds has been attempted by incubation of membranes isolated from rat adipocytes and liver in the presence of concentrations of DTT as high as 50 mM. Even this high concentration of reductant does not dissociate the native insulin receptor in membranes beyond the partially reduced ($\alpha\beta$) state as determined by SDS-PAGE.

The high resistance of Class II disulfide bonds to reduction is not solely due to these sites in the receptor structure being protected by the membrane bilayer; a similar resistance to DTT is observed when the membranes are solubilized in the non-ionic detergent Triton X-100 before treatment with reductant. Hence, their resistance is most likely due to a key disulfide bridge(s) in a particular domain of the ($\alpha\beta$) complex not available for interaction with DTT. This domain becomes exposed when the insulin receptor is solubilized and denatured in SDS[17,27]. Under these conditions a low concentration of DTT will reduce Class I disulfide bridges, as depicted in Fig. 2 (Reaction 2). High concentrations of DTT in the presence of SDS split the Class II disulfides, releasing the free α and β insulin receptor subunits (Reaction 3).

The integrity of the Class I disulfide bridges in the ($\alpha\beta$)$_2$ insulin receptor complex is not essential for insulin binding. As described above, the free ($\alpha\beta$) receptor halves will bind ^{125}I-insulin and the halves can be affinity-labelled and visualized on gels. Furthermore, twice as much ^{125}I-insulin binds to rat adipocytes when the receptors are dissociated into ($\alpha\beta$) halves. The ($\alpha\beta$) halves do not appear to become physically dissociated when the disulfide bridges linking them are reduced. When adipocyte membranes containing partially reduced ($\alpha\beta$) receptor complexes are solubilized in Triton X-100 and treated with a cross-linking agent, a receptor complex of Mr 350,000 ($\alpha\beta$)$_2$ resistant to reduction in SDS can be obtained (Massague and Czech, unpublished). This suggests that at least some of the ($\alpha\beta$) receptor halves generated by DTT remain closely associated by non-covalent interactions even after detergent-dispersion of the membrane structures, and can be irreversibly cross-linked under the above conditions. Native ($\alpha\beta$) receptor fragments have been

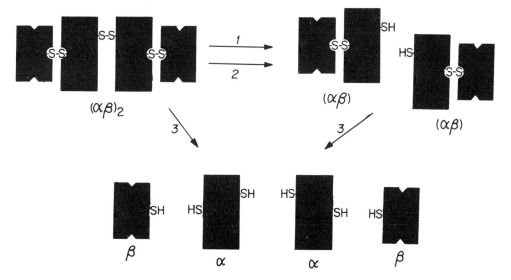

1- Non-denatured, 1-10 mM DTT
2- Denatured, low reductant (0.5mM DTT)
3- Denatured, high reductant (5 mM DTT)

Fig. 2. Reduction of the insulin receptor. The insulin receptor contains two classes of disulfide bridges that differ in their sensitivity to reductants. The highest sensitivity is exhibited by the disulfide linkage(s) between the two symmetrical ($\alpha\beta$) halves of the molecule[17,31,32]. *The individual α and β subunits are dissociated from the complex under stringent reduction conditions after denaturation in SDS.*

detected in membrane preparations from rat liver and other tissues under conditions where exogenous reduction was absent[26]. The physiological role of different redox states of the insulin receptor in plasma membranes may be important for insulin action and/or receptor regulation.

A unique proteolytic cleavage site on the β subunit

The native, $(\alpha\beta)_2$, insulin receptor in the cell surface of intact rat adipocytes, and presumably of many other kinds of cells, contains a site on each of the two β subunits that is particularly sensitive to certain cellular and exogenous proteases[17,27]. This property has greatly facilitated the elucidation of the exact subunit stoichiometry of the insulin receptor disulfide-linked complexes.

Specific proteolytic processing can excise a portion of each β subunit of the $(\alpha\beta)_2$ receptor complex, leaving a fragment of Mr 49,000, (the β_1 receptor subunit fragment) disulfide-linked to the receptor core. This process can affect the two β subunits sequentially; the $(\alpha\beta)_2$ (Mr 350,000) native receptor form being transformed first into a $(\alpha\beta)(\alpha\beta_1)$ (Mr 320,000) and then into a $(\alpha\beta_1)_2$ (Mr 290,000) receptor state (Fig. 3). Partially purified membranes from all tissues examined contain these three receptor forms which are readily resolved by affinity labeling, SDS-electrophoresis and autoradiography of the electrophoretic gels. It is not clear whether the β_2 fragment remains associated with the receptor complex in the native membrane.

Mild reduction of the corresponding Class I disulfide bridges splits the $(\alpha\beta)_2$ and the $(\alpha\beta_1)_2$ receptor forms into $(\alpha\beta)$ (Mr 210,000) and $(\alpha\beta_1)$ (Mr 160,000) partially reduced halves, respectively. Denaturation and extreme reducing conditions dissociate these halves into the corresponding α and β or β_1 receptor subunits. In contrast, the mild reduction of the $(\alpha\beta)(\alpha\beta_1)$ receptor form generates the two different sized partially reduced $(\alpha\beta)$ and $(\alpha\beta_1)$ fragments that can be resolved electrophoretically. The complete reduction of these two fragments excised separately from electrophoretic gels generates α and β or α and β_1 receptor subunits, respectively. Thus, the unique asymmetry of the $(\alpha\beta)$ $(\alpha\beta_1)$ insulin receptor form means that each partially or totally reduced species derived from it can be distinguished in SDS-polyacrylamide gels. Such studies on the sequential reduction of this asymmetrical form of the insulin receptor elucidated the precise subunit stoichiometry of this and other receptor forms[17].

The precursor-product relationship between the β and the β_1 receptor subunit species is suggested by multiple similarities in their respective peptide maps[27]. The endogenous source of proteolytic activity that acts to 'nick' the β subunit is apparently the lysosomes. Incubation of plasma membranes with a lysosomal fraction from rat adipocytes remarkably increases the ratio of the $(\alpha\beta)(\alpha\beta_1)$ and $(\alpha\beta_1)_2$ forms in the membrane[27]. Affinity-labeled membranes from rat adipocytes incubated with the lysosomotropic agent chloroquine before cell homogenization have fewer proteolytically-transformed receptor forms (Pilch, Axelrod and Czech, unpublished). Plasma membranes themselves do not seem to contain any proteolytic activity capable of catalyzing the conversion of the β to β_1 subunit[27].

The proteolytic nature of the β subunit transformation and the topography of the sensitive sites have been further confirmed by elastase-treatment of the native $(\alpha\beta)_2$ receptor on the cell surface of intact adipocytes[29]. This protease, but not trypsin, α-chymotrypsin or *Staphylococcus aureus* V$_8$ protease, catalyzed the limited proteolysis of the β subunit, transforming the $(\alpha\beta)_2$ receptor form successively into the $(\alpha\beta)(\alpha\beta_1)$ and $(\alpha\beta_1)_2$ forms. These experiments showed that the protease-sensitive site is on the extracellular face of the receptor structure. The presence of variable amounts of β and β_1 subunits in preparations of plasma membranes and purified receptor reported by various laboratories is most likely due to a variable degree of membrane-lysosomal interaction during the isolation of these samples. Nevertheless, the possibility that the $(\alpha\beta)(\alpha\beta_1)$ and $(\alpha\beta_1)_2$ receptor forms are natural components of the intact cell cannot be ruled out as they may well be the initial products in the *in vivo* lysosomal processing of the $(\alpha\beta)_2$ receptor form.

Structure-function relationships and receptor conformation

In many previous studies of insulin binding and action the receptor may have been heterogeneous. It was therefore interesting to examine these parameters under conditions of defined receptor structure. Elastase-treated fat cells, bearing the $(\alpha\beta_1)_2$ receptor, exhibit the same sensitivity to insulin as untreated cells in their ability to elevate glucose oxidation in response to the hormone[29]. Both treated and untreated cells also bind insulin with essentially the same affinity (Kd = 3×10^{-9}M) and maximal binding capacity (200 fmol/10^6 cells). Therefore, receptor heterogeneity does not seem to seriously complicate studies of insulin binding and action.

A proteolytically altered receptor can also be generated by treating adipocytes with trypsin. Trypsin exhibits an insulin-like action in increasing the rate of glucose oxidation in adipocytes in rough correlation with its proteolytic fragmentation of the intact receptor[33]. However, after trypsinization of cells has partially stimulated glucose oxidation and cleaved the insulin receptor into several fragments, the sensitivity of the trypsin-treated cells to a further insulin-mediated stimulation of hexose oxidation is identical to untreated

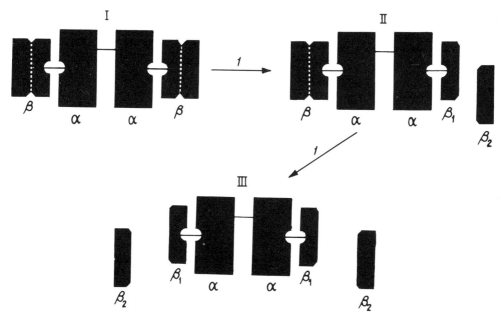

1-Lysosomal protease(s), Elastase

Fig. 3. Generation of three ubiquitous insulin receptor forms by a proteolytic fragmentation of the β subunit. Receptor forms I, II, and III are present in membrane preparations in all tissues studied and can be readily resolved in SDS gels (apparent mol. wts 350,000, 320,000 and 290,000, respectively)[17]*. The native 350,000 receptor can be sequentially converted to the 320,000 and 290,000 forms in vitro by elastase*[27].

adipocytes[33]. This proteolysis increases the affinity of the receptors but decreases their number. Thus, at any given hormone concentration the number of receptors occupied is similar to control cells. Insulin action can therefore be mediated by a receptor that has undergone substantial proteolytic cleavage. We suggest that the receptor remains intact in essentially its native quaternary structure despite breakage of some peptide bonds in the amino acid sequence. Interestingly, it was reported that all four subunits of the acetylcholine receptor can be extensively 'nicked' by papain, but the receptor retains full functional activity even when only fragments of one subunit are evident in SDS-gels[34].

The detailed way in which insulin binds to its receptor and elicits its various biological responses is not known. It is assumed however that hormone binding triggers a change in receptor structure leading to a transmembrane signal. Consistent with this notion is our recent demonstration that the occupied α receptor subunit is more sensitive to tryptic digestion than the unoccupied receptor[35]. This indicates that the insulin receptor α subunits undergo a ligand-induced conformational change which may be requisite for insulin action. Alternatively, the hormone may stabilize a receptor conformation that is normally in equilibrium with other receptor states.

Subunit composition of other polypeptide hormone and growth factor receptors

A number of polypeptide hormones and/or growth factors such as nerve growth factor (NGF), multiplication stimulating activity (MSA), insulin-like growth factors (IGFs), and relaxin show considerable sequence homology with insulin[36]. Some of these growth factors exhibit insulin-like biological activity and there exists some degree of mutual competition for receptor binding. There is, therefore, considerable interest in identifying the respective receptors from a structural and evolutionary point of view. Using the same affinity cross-linking techniques and reagents employed to label the insulin receptor, a MSA receptor has been linked to ^{125}I-MSA in membranes from rat liver, fat and human placenta[37]. This MSA receptor migrates in SDS-gels as a single band of Mr 265,000 when affinity-labeled membranes from these tissues are solubilized in SDS and DTT. When DTT is omitted the apparent mol. wt of the receptor is 225,000, indicating the presence of considerable intrachain disulfide bonds. Thus, the MSA-binding protein differs in size and lacks the disulfide-linked subunit structure seen for the insulin receptor, but both receptors do appear to possess intrachain disulfide linkages. The lack of covalently linked subunits in this MSA receptor does not rule out a more complex non-covalent subunit structure which is completely dissociated by our SDS-PAGE analyses. In very recent experiments we have affinity-labeled an IGF-I receptor in human skin fibroblast and placenta membranes that contains a subunit composition and stoichiometry similar to that of the insulin receptor (Massague and Czech, manuscript in preparation). We are currently employing affinity cross-linking techniques to investigate the comparative biochemistry of these and other growth factor receptors.

Conclusion

Structural information, albeit rudimentary, is now available about insulin receptor subunits and their disposition within the receptor complex. The $(\alpha\beta)_2$ disulfide-linked receptor structure proposed here is consistent with a large body of data from various laboratories. In addition to the α and β subunits identified by affinity-labeling, other unlabeled receptor subunits may, of course, be present. Such subunits, possibly loosely bound to the receptor complex, may be released from the structure during affinity purification in detergent solution. Further efforts will be required to confirm or eliminate this possibility. In any case, the framework for such further investigation and for more detailed structural work on the α and β subunits is now in place.

The key unresolved issue about the insulin receptor relates to the immediate and specific biological activity in which it participates. The structural aspects of the insulin receptor now revealed do not yet solve this central mystery. We need to understand whether the receptor has catalytic capability analogous to an enzyme, or whether it might serve as an effector or substrate in an enzymic reaction or cascade. This question may be difficult to answer if the complex environment of the native cell surface membrane needs to be intact for us to observe receptor function. Our new knowledge of the structure of insulin receptors has been extremely useful, but we may need new methods to find out the molecular details of insulin receptor function.

Acknowledgements

The work performed by the authors and cited in this review was supported by NIH grants AM 17893 and AM 27027 and a grant from the Kroc Foundation. We wish to thank Sandy Brenner for excellent secretarial assistance.

References

1 Czech, M. (1980) *Diabetes* 29, 399–409
2 Kahn, R. C. (1979) *Trends Biochem. Sci.* 263–266
3 Hepp, K. D. (1977) *Diabetologia* 13, 177
4 Czech, M. P. (1977) *Ann. Rev. Biochem.* 46, 359–384
5 Czech, M. P. (1981) *Am. J. Med.* 70, 142–150
6 Roth, J., Kahn, C. R., Lesniak, M. A., Gorden, P., DeMeyts, P., Megyesi, K., Neville, D. M. Jr., Gavin, J. E., III, Soll, A. H., Freychet, P., Goldfine, I. D., Bar, R. S., Archer, J. A. (1975) *Recent Prog. Horm. Res.* 31, 95–139
7 Guatrecasas, P. (1972) *Proc. Natl. Acad. Sci. U.S.A.* 69, 1277–1281
8 Kono, T., Barham, F. W., (1971) *J. Biol. Chem.* 246, 6210–6216
9 Caro, J. F., Amatruda, J. M. (1980) *J. Biol. Chem.* 255, 10052–10055
10 Terris, S., Steiner, D. F. (1975) *J. Biol. Chem.* 250, 8389–8389
11 Gavin, J. R. III, Roth, R., Neville, D. M. Jr., DeMeyts, P., Buell, D. N. (1974) *Proc. Natl. Acad. Sci. U.S.A.* 71, 84–88
12 Archer, J. A., Gorden, P., Roth, J. (1976) *J. Clin. Invest.* 55, 166–174
13 Olefsky, J. M. (1976) *J. Clin. Invest.* 57, 842–851
14 Marshall, S., Olefsky, J. M. (1979) *J. Biol. Chem.* 254, 10153–10160
15 Muggeo, M., VanObberghen, E., Kahn, C. R., Roth, J., Ginsberg, B. H., DeMeyts, P., Emdin, S. O., Falkmer, S. (1979) *Diabetes* 28, 175–181
16 Jacobs, S., Schechter, Y., Bissell, K., Cuatrecasas, P. (1977) *Biochem. Biophys. Res. Comm.* 981–988
17 Massague, J., Pilch, P. F., Czech, M. P. (1980) *Proc. Natl. Acad. Sci. U.S.A.*, 77, 7137–7141
18 Yip, C. C., Yeung, C. W. T., Moule, M. L. (1978) *J. Biol. Chem.* 253, 1743–1745
19 Yip, C. C., Yeung, C. W. T., Moule, M. L. (1980) *Biochemistry* 19, 70–76
20 Yeung, C. W. T., Moule, M. L., Yip, C. C. (1980) *Biochemistry* 19, 2196–2203
21 Pilch, P. F., Czech, M. P. (1979) *J. Biol. Chem.* 254, 3375–3381
22 Pilch, P. F., Czech, M. P. (1980) *J. Biol. Chem.* 255, 1722–1731
23 Heinrich, J., Pilch, P. F., Czech, M. P. (1980) *J. Biol. Chem.* 255, 1732–1737
24 Lang, Y. Kahn, C. R., Harrison, L. C. (1980) *Biochemistry* 19, 64–70
25 Harrison, L. C., Itin, A. (1980) *J. Biol. Chem.* 255, 12066–12072
26 Massague, J., Czech, M. P. (1980) *Diabetes* 29, 945–947
27 Massague, J., Pilch, P. F., Czech, M. P. (1981) *J. Biol. Chem.* 256, 3182–3190
28 Jacobs, S., Hazum, E., Cuatrecasas (1980) *J. Biol. Chem.* 255, 6937–6940
29 Pilch, P. F., Czech, M. P. (1980) *Serono Symposia Series* (in press)
30 Jacobs, S., Hazum, E., Cuatrecasas (1980) *Biochem. Biophys. Res. Comm.* 94, 1066–1073
31 Jacobs, S., Hazum, E., Schnechter, Y., Cuatrecasas, P. (1979) *Proc. Natl. Acad. Sci. U.S.A.* 76, 4918–4921
32 Massague, J., Czech, M. P. (1980) *Serono Symposia Series* (in press)
33 Pilch, P. F., Azelrod, J. D., Colello, J., Czech, M. P. (1981) *J. Biol. Chem.*, 256, 1570–1575
34 Lindstrom, J., Gullick, W., Conti-Tronconi, B., Ellisman, M. (1980) *Biochemistry* 19, 4791–4795
35 Pilch, P. F., Czech, M. P. (1980) *Science* 210, 1152–1153
36 Bradshaw, R. A., Niall, H. D. (1978) *Trends Biochem. Sci.* 3, 274–278
37 Massague, J., Guillette, B. J., Czech, M. P. (1981) *J. Biol. Chem.*, 256, 2122–2125

Does phosphatidylinositol breakdown control the Ca^{2+}-gating mechanism?

S. Cockcroft

Department of Experimental Pathology, School of Medicine, University College London, University Street, London WC1E 6JJ, U.K.

A cell-surface receptor specifically recognizes its ligand and this initiates a train of events which culminates in the functional response of the cell. Transmission of information into the cell interior occurs via increased intracellular concentrations of second messengers such as cAMP or Ca^{2+}. The sequence of molecular events that leads to elevation of cAMP is fairly well understood but this is not the case for Ca^{2+}. One biochemical event which has been suggested to play a key role in controlling a rise in cytosolic Ca^{2+} is breakdown of phosphatidylinositol (PI), a quantitatively minor anionic phospholipid. Metabolic turnover of PI is stimulated by many cell-surface receptors when they interact with their appropriate ligands. Table I shows a selected sample of cell types and ligands that are known to induce changes in PI turnover as well as triggering functional responses such as exocytosis, contraction or proliferation.

The initial step in PI turnover is the breakdown of PI, which is followed by its resynthesis. A Ca^{2+}-dependent phospholipase C, specific for PI, catalyses its breakdown into diacylglycerol and inositol-phosphates. The diacylglycerol is rapidly phosphorylated to form phosphatidic acid which is converted back into PI with CDP-diacylglycerol as an intermediate (Fig. 1).

Michell[1], in 1975, made an interesting finding that PI metabolism is triggered only by those receptors that control a rise in cytosolic Ca^{2+} which then acts as the second messenger for stimulating the functional response of the cell. Receptors that stimulate adenylate cyclase do not show changes in PI metabolism. He went further and observed that enhanced PI metabolism triggered in a number of cell types did not appear to be dependent on the rise in cytosolic Ca^{2+} whereas the functional response was. The observation was largely based on four different lines of evidence. (1) Removal of Ca^{2+} from the external medium abolished the functional response but not PI turnover. (2) Introduction of Ca^{2+} into the cell with an ionophore provoked the functional response but not PI turnover. (3) A class of drugs one of whose actions is to antagonize the stimulated entry of Ca^{2+} into cells did not affect PI metabolism but abolished the functional response. (4) Dose–response relationships showed that PI metabolism closely follows the extent of receptor occupancy rather than the functional response. All this circumstantial evidence suggested that PI breakdown (the crucial step in the process) precedes the entry of Ca^{2+} into cells and could therefore be a universal biochemical event intrinsic to the Ca^{2+}-gating mechanism[1,2]. A virtue of this suggestion is that it is predictive and at the same time imposes certain restrictions which makes it testable. Firstly, it is predicted that stimulated breakdown of PI will be found to be a response of all Ca^{2+}-mobilizing receptors, and of no other type of receptor. Secondly, PI breakdown must be a consequence of receptor occupancy and not of Ca^{2+} mobilization

Evidence from a number of cell types examined since the original list of tissues was compiled in 1975 has generally supported the hypothesis. Not only has no receptor known to control other second messengers (e.g. cAMP) been shown to stimulate turnover of PI, but the correlation between PI turnover and Ca^{2+}-mobilizing receptors has been considerably extended (e.g. mast cells, hepatocytes, lacrimal gland, blowfly salivary gland and various smooth muscles). However, in the last year, evidence has appeared from a number of sources which now suggests that PI breakdown is not universally a Ca^{2+}-independent phenomenon.

The philosopher of science, Karl Popper, has pointed out that any hypothesis is refuted when falsified by one event. For example, if one has only ever seen white swans then one speculates that all swans are white. The discovery of one black swan falsifies the hypothesis. In the context of this discussion, any example of Ca^{2+}-dependent PI turnover will resemble the 'black swan'.

This article will look at the Ca^{2+} sensitivity of PI turnover in a number of systems to assess the validity of the hypothesis that PI breakdown is the universal biochemical event that controls the Ca^{2+}-gating mechanism.

Ca^{2+} sensitivity of stimulated PI metabolism

There are at least 30 different cell types in which stimulation of Ca^{2+}-mobilizing receptors induces enhanced turnover of PI. The Ca^{2+} sensitivity of PI turnover has not always been assessed and Table I summarizes the available information. The role of Ca^{2+} in PI metabolism in neutrophils and platelets will be discussed in detail with a brief look at other systems for comparison.

Neutrophils show a multiplicity of functions when stimulated with soluble agonists such as f-metleuphe, a synthetic tripeptide mimicking bacterial factors. This stimulates chemotaxis and low level secretion of lysosomal enzymes. Addition of cytochalisin B represses the chemotactic response and potentiates secretion, which thus becomes an easily quantified measure of cell function. The f-metleuphe receptor of neutrophils is a Ca^{2+}-mobilizing receptor which stimulates turnover of PI. (PI turnover is not dependent on cytochalisin B.) Secretion by neutrophils is rapid, but since PI breakdown occurs within 10 s of addition of the ligand it would be a sufficiently early response to participate in the Ca^{2+}-gating mechanism.

F-metleuphe stimulation triggers both PI breakdown and optimal secretion from neutrophils in the presence of external Ca^{2+}. In the absence of external Ca^{2+}, se-

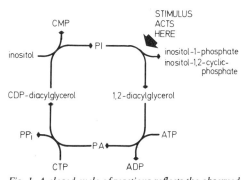

Fig. 1. A closed cycle of reactions reflects the observed changes in phosphatidylinositol metabolism. PI turnover has generally been studied either by measuring chemical or radiochemical breakdown of PI (the primary event) or by incorporation of radioactive precursors ($^{32}P_i$ or [^3H]inositol) into PI (secondary event). PA, phosphatidic acid.

cretion occurs at a lower level and this is supported by mobilization of an internal pool of Ca^{2+}. The effect of Ca^{2+} removal on PI turnover, however, is to abolish the breakdown and the consequent resynthesis of PI. If Ca^{2+} is introduced into the cell with an ionophore, thus by-passing the receptor, neutrophils respond by secreting lysosomal enzymes and also by breaking down PI[3,4]. Therefore, in neutrophils, it is the entry of Ca^{2+} into the cytosol which causes PI breakdown.

Like neutrophils, platelets show a multiplicity of responses such as shape change, aggregation and secretion. Mobilization of Ca^{2+} in platelets is from intracellular stores, which can also be utilized by a Ca^{2+} ionophore. Breakdown of PI is stimulated by thrombin within 10 s and a transient rise in diacylglycerol followed by the appearance of phosphatidic acid and PI has been observed. The Ca^{2+} ionophore is also capable of stimulating PI breakdown. Moreover, the effects of thrombin and ionophore are not additive, indicating that both stimuli utilize the same pool of PI[5]. Alterations in the availability of Ca^{2+} can be achieved in a variety of ways in platelets. Additions of the Ca^{2+} chelator, EGTA, or an inhibitor of intracellular Ca^{2+} translocation, TMB-8, leads to inhibition of platelet function and also PI breakdown. Both effects of TMB-8 can be reversed by addition of external Ca^{2+}. Increased levels of

TABLE I. Sensitivity of PI response to Ca^{2+}

Tissue	Agonist	PI response sensitive to Ca^{2+} ext	PI response triggered with Ca^{2+} ionophore
I. Ca^{2+} is the only stimulus			
Neutrophils	F-metleuphe	Yes	Yes
Lymphocytes[13,14]	Phytohaemagluttinin	Yes	Yes
Mast cells	ATP^{4-}	Yes	Yes
Platelets	Thrombin	No*	Yes
Pancreas[17]	Acetylcholine	Yes	Yes
II. Either Ca^{2+} or receptor occupancy is the stimulus			
Vas deferens[15]	Acetylcholine	No	Yes
Thyroid	Acetylcholine	No	Yes
Mast cells	Con A, antigen	No	Yes
Hepatocytes	Angiotensin	Partial	No
Synaptosomes	Acetylcholine	Yes	?
Iris smooth muscle	Noradrenaline	Partial	?
Ileum smooth muscle	Carbamoylcholine	Partial	?
III. Receptor occupancy is the sole stimulus			
Blowfly salivary gland	5-hydroxytryptamine	No	No
Parotid	Acetylcholine	No	No
Adrenal medulla	Acetylcholine	No	?
Lacrimal gland	Acetyl-β-methylcholine	No	?
Anterior pituitary	Acetylcholine	No	?

* See text.
Complete citation can be found in Ref. 3 except where indicated.

cAMP antagonize Ca^{2+} mobilization and hence platelet function, and also inhibit the changes in PI metabolism[6]. Thus, in platelets Ca^{2+} is likely to be the trigger of PI breakdown.

The mast cells show anomalous behaviour. Secretion of histamine from mast cells stimulated with Con A or ATP^{4-} requires external Ca^{2+}. Changes in PI metabolism, though triggered by either stimulus, show differences in their Ca^{2+} requirements. While Con A-stimulated PI turnover is independent of external Ca^{2+}, ATP^{4-}-induced PI turnover is Ca^{2+} dependent[7,8]. Also the ionophore is effective in stimulating PI metabolism[9]. The contrasting behaviour of different mast cell receptors suggests that PI metabolism can be controlled by two separate routes. In one case, Ca^{2+} itself is the trigger and, in the same cell, occupation of a receptor can be a sufficient stimulus to trigger PI metabolism.

At the other end of the spectrum are a number of cell types where Ca^{2+} entry alone will not stimulate PI turnover. Receptor occupancy is the sole stimulus in these cells. Examples are the parotid gland and blowfly salivary gland where addition of Ca^{2+} ionophore does not trigger PI turnover.

Table I summarizes the varying effects of Ca^{2+} on PI metabolism in those cell types where the question has been addressed. These fall roughly into three groups. The first group where Ca^{2+} alone is the stimulus, the second group where Ca^{2+} or occupancy of the receptor can be a trigger and the third group where receptor occupancy is the sole stimulus.

Possible functions of PI metabolism

Although PI breakdown cannot play a direct role in the Ca^{2+}-gating mechanism originally envisaged[1], the provocative correlation between Ca^{2+}-mobilizing receptors and PI breakdown still holds good. So, what can be its function?

A recent proposal based on studies on platelets suggests that PI could be a source of arachidonic acid for the synthesis of prostaglandins, thromboxanes and other arachidonic acid-derived metabolites[5]. (PI has a distinct fatty acid composition in that the acyl group in the second position is predominantly arachidonic acid.) Various observations militate against this possibility. (1) The amount of PI broken down is compensated by a quantitive increase in phosphatidic acid (or diacylglycerol, or both) in two cell-types where this point has been studied[6,10]. (2) All tissues which show enhanced PI turnover are not necessarily major sources of arachidonic acid-derived metabolites. For example, pancreas produces only 277 pmol of prostaglandins per gram of tissue whilst the amount of PI broken down is 174 nmol per gram of tissue, a difference of 3 orders of magnitude[11]. (3) In some tissues, arachidonic acid-derived metabolites exceed the amount of PI present. Macrophages, in which 25% of the total fatty acids are arachidonic acid, can mobilize 50% of their total arachidonic acid content. Since PI only constitutes 6% of the total cell phospholipid it cannot be the major source[12]. (4) In a number of tissues (e.g. platelets, fibroblasts, neutrophils and macrophages) phosphatidylcholine and phosphatidylethanolamine lose arachidonic acid on stimulation suggesting that these phospholipids are probably the main source.

What are the other common denominators that Ca^{2+}-mobilizing receptors would possess? One that readily springs to mind is the control of intracellular Ca^{2+} after receptor stimulation. Levels of Ca^{2+} within the cell are finely regulated and it is possible that the breakdown of PI has a role to play in the removal of Ca^{2+} from the cell. Another possibility is desensitization. This occurs at two levels; desensitization of the specific receptor and general desensitization of the whole cell. It may be relevant that according to the cell type, PI breakdown can be controlled either by receptor occupancy, or at the level of cytosolic Ca^{2+}, or both.

To conclude, there is a close relationship between cell activation of Ca^{2+}-mobilizing receptors and the stimulation of PI metabolism. However, the hypothesis that PI breakdown is a reaction intrinsic to the Ca^{2+}-gating mechanism is negated by the recent sightings of 'black swans'. Receptor-stimulated PI breakdown is still a response in search of a role.

Acknowledgements

I would like to thank Drs J. P. Bennett and B. D. Gomperts (Department of Experimental Pathology, University College, London) for reading the manuscript. This work was supported by the Wellcome Trust.

Reading list

1 Michell, R. H. (1975) *Biochim. Biophys. Acta* 415, 81–147
2 Michell, R. H. and Kirk, C. J. (1981) *Trends Pharmacol. Sci.* 2, 86–89
3 Cockcroft, S., Bennett, J. P. and Gomperts, B. D. (1980) *FEBS Lett.* 110, 115–118
4 Cockcroft, S., Bennett, J. P. and Gomperts, B. D. (1980) *Nature (London)* 288, 275–277
5 Bell, R. L. and Majerus, P. W. (1980) *J. Biol. Chem.* 255, 1790–1792
6 Broekman, M., Ward, J. W. and Marcus, A. J. (1980) *J. Clin. Invest.* 66, 275–283
7 Cockcroft, S. and Gomperts, B. D. (1979) *Biochem. J.* 178, 681–687
8 Cockcroft, S. and Gomperts, B. D. (1980) *Biochem. J.* 188, 789–798
9 Kennerly, D. A., Sullivan, T. J. and Parker, C. W. (1979) *J. Immunol.* 122, 152–159
10 Geison, R. L., Banschbach, M. W., Sadeghian, K. and Hokin-Neaverson, M. (1976) *Biochem. Biophys. Res. Comm.* 68, 343–349
11 Banschbach, M. W. and Hokin-Neaverson, M. (1980) *FEBS Lett.* 177, 131–133
12 Scott, W. A., Zrike, J. M., Hamill, A. L., Kempe, J. and Cohn. Z. A. (1980) *J. Exp. Med.* 152, 324–335
13 Hui, O. Y. and Harmony, K. A. K. (1980) *Biochem. J.* 192, 91–98
14 Allan, D. and Michell, R. H. (1977) *Biochem. J.* 164, 389–397
15 Egawa, K., Sacktor, B. and Takenawa, T. (1981) *Biochem. J.* 194, 129–136
16 Haye, B., Marcy, G. and Jacquemin, C. (1979) *Biochimie* 61, 905–912
17 Farese, R. V., Larson, R. E. and Sabir, M. A. (1980) *Biochim. Biophys. Acta* 633, 479–484

Phospholipid methylation and the receptor-induced release of histamine from cells

Julius Axelrod and Fusao Hirata

Section on Pharmacology, Laboratory of Clinical Science, National Institute of Mental Health, Bethesda, MD 20205, U.S.A.

A major problem in pharmacology is how biochemical signals in the form of neurotransmitters, hormones, drugs and antibodies transmit their messages through cell membranes. In the past few years our laboratory has observed that methylation of phospholipids plays an important role in the transduction of biochemical signals through membranes. We have found that rat mast cells and basophilic leukemia cells have served as productive models to study membrane lipid methylation in the receptor-mediated release of histamine.

Upon suitable stimulation, histamine is released from mast cells and basophils by a process of exocytosis requiring two steps. In the first, receptors on the membrane are activated by an antigen. In the second, granules containing histamine fuse with the plasma membrane and the amines are then displaced from their binding site and released to the exterior of the cell[1]. Mast cells have specific receptors on their surface which interact with IgE and its antigens as well as lectins, such as concanavalin A (Con A)[2]. This interaction then initiates a series of complex changes in the cell which ultimately leads to the release of histamine. During the past few years our laboratory, in collaboration with those of the Ishizakas at Johns Hopkins and Siraganian at the NIH, has shown that the receptor-mediated release of histamine involves phospholipid methylation, phospholipase A_2 activation and arachidonic acid release.

We have found that many receptor-mediated events lead to the conversion of phosphatidylethanolamine to phosphatidylcholine by transmethylation reactions. Two methyltransferase enzymes are involved in the formation of phosphatidylcholine as follows:

phosphatidylethanolamine (PE) $\xrightarrow{\text{PMT I}}$ phosphatidyl-N-monomethylethanolamine (PMM) $\xrightarrow[+ 2\,CH_3]{\text{PMT II}}$ phosphatidylcholine (PC)[3].

S-adenosylmethionine (SAM) serves as the methyl donor for both reactions. The first reaction requires Mg^{2+} and has a low K_m for SAM; the second has a much higher K_m for SAM and does not require Mg^{2+}. In red cell membranes, liver microsomes and possibly other cell membranes, PE is translocated from the cytoplasmic side of the membrane to the outer surface as it is successively methylated to phosphatidylcholine (Fig. 1). In the course of the flip-flop of the methylated phospholipids, the

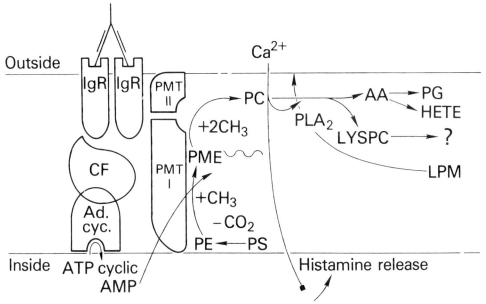

Fig. 1. IgE mediated phospholipid cascade and histamine release. IgE Receptor (IgR), phospholipid methyltransferase I (PMT I), phospholipid methyltransferase II (PMT II), phosphatidylserine (PS), phosphatidylethanolamine (PE), phosphatidyl-N-monomethylethanolamine (PME), phosphatidylcholine (PC), phospholipase A_2 (PLA$_2$), arachidonic acid (AA), prostaglandin (PG), lysophosphatidylcholine (LYSPC), 12-L-hydroxy-5,8,10,14-eicosatetraenoic acid (HETE), lipomodulin (LPM), a phospholipase A_2 inhibitory protein[12], coupling factor (CF), adenylate cyclase (Ad cyc) and change in fluidity ($\sim\!\sim$).

membrane viscosity is reduced[3]. Changes in membrane viscosity due to methylation affect lateral mobility and coupling of β-adrenergic receptors with adenylate cyclase[3].

In initial experiments studying the release of histamine in rat mast cells we observed that stimulation with Con A in the presence of phosphatidylserine, Mg^{2+} and Ca^{2+} gave a transient increase of phospholipid methylation followed by release of histamine[3]. Subsequent experiments using ^{14}C-labeled phosphatidylserine showed that upon treatment of mast cells with Con A, phosphatidylserine was converted to PE by decarboxylation which was then methylated to PC. The latter compound was further metabolized by removal of a fatty acid to lysophosphatidylcholine as follows:

phosphatidylserine (PS) $\xrightarrow{-CO_2}$ phosphatidylethanolamine (PE) $\xrightarrow{+CH_3}$ phosphatidyl-N-monomethylethanolamine (PMM) $\xrightarrow{+2CH_3}$ phosphatidylcholine (PC) $\xrightarrow{-\text{fatty acid}}$ lysophosphatidylcholine. Mg^{2+} was shown to be required for phospholipid methylation and Ca^{2+} for histamine release.

Mast cell histamine release is initiated by bridging surface receptors by divalent Con A lectin. Recent work has shown that in chicken erythrocytes, divalent, but not monovalent, Con A stimulates both phospholipid methylation and membrane fluidity[4]. Mast cells have specific receptors for IgE. When IgE molecules on the cell surface are cross-linked with either multivalent antigens or divalent antibodies to IgE, histamine is released in a non-cytotoxic manner[2]. By bridging the IgE receptor with antibody (anti-RBL) or its F(ab')$_2$ fragment, histamine is released without the participation of IgE. Binding of monovalent F(ab') fragments of the antibody to the IgE receptor antibody does not release the amine[5].

To examine the role of phospholipid methylation in the receptor-mediated release of histamine, mast cells were first incubated with [^{3}H]methylmethionine, [^{3}H]Methionine is rapidly converted to S-adenosyl-[^{3}H]methyl-L-methionine and this is followed by the transfer of the [^{3}H] methyl group to phospholipids, mainly phosphatidylcholine[5]. The addition of anti-RBL caused a transient increase in the incorporation of [^{3}H]methyl group into phospholipids. Maximal transfer of the methyl group takes place in 10–15 s followed by a fall to base-line values by 30 s. To see whether the bridging of the IgE receptors was necessary for increased phospholipid methylation, as is the case for histamine release, mast cells were incubated with [^{3}H]methionine and challenged with either F(ab')$_2$ or F(ab') monomer fragments of anti-RBL. F(ab')$_2$, but not F(ab'), fragments induced a rapid and transient increase in the incorporation of a methyl group into phospholipids.

As in many secretory processes Ca^{2+} is also required for the release of histamine in mast cells. Stimulation of mast cells with anti-RBL or its F(ab')$_2$ fragments caused an influx of Ca^{2+} into these cells. Maximum influx of Ca^{2+} occurred within 2 min shortly followed by the release of histamine. Phospholipid methylation preceded these processes. The association of IgE receptor-mediated phospholipid methylation, Ca^{2+} influx and histamine release was examined by the use of methyltransferase inhibitors. Compounds such as 3-deaza-adenosine (3-DZA) or S-isobutyryl-3-deaza-adenosine (3-deaza-SIBA) can enter cells and then form metabolites that inhibit methyltransferase reactions[6]. The effect of methyltransferase inhibitors on receptor-mediated phospholipid methylations, Ca^{2+} influx and histamine released was examined. [^{3}H]methyl group incorporated into phospholipids, Ca^{2+} influx and histamine release were all inhibited to a similar degree in a dose-dependent manner by the methyltransferase inhibitors after stimulation with anti-RBL[5]. All of these experiments indicated that there is a close association among the IgE receptor, phospholipid methylation, Ca^{2+} influx and histamine release (Fig. 1).

Many investigations have shown that stimulation of an antigen-induced release of histamine in mast cells is inhibited after increasing the levels of cyclic AMP. Stimulation of mast cells with F(ab')$_2$ fragments of anti-RBL causes a transient increase in cyclic AMP reaching a maximum level at about 30 s. This prompted a study on the relationship of the stimulatory effect of phospholipid methylation on histamine release and its inhibition by cyclic AMP[7]. Mast cells were incubated with [^{3}H]methionine and theophylline. Theophylline is a compound that inhibits phosphodiesterase and this blocks the metabolism of cyclic AMP. The addition of theophylline causes an increase in cyclic AMP and a decreased methylation of lipids, influx of Ca^{2+} and histamine release after stimulation of mast cells with anti-RBL. In additional experiments to show the relationship between cyclic AMP and lipid methylation mast cell plasma membranes were isolated. When membranes were treated with F(ab')$_2$ fragments of anti-RBL there was an increased formation of cyclic AMP[7]. There was also an increase in phospholipid methylation in these treated membranes. When S-adenosyl-[^{3}H]methyl-L-methionine was added, monovalent F(ab') had no effect on cyclic AMP or phospholipid methylation. The addition of dibutyryl cyclic AMP to membranes also blocked the increase in phospholipid methylation when the IgE receptor was stimulated. These results suggest that the IgE receptor is linked to both the methyltransferase enzymes and adenylate cyclase (Fig. 1). Methyltransferases probably serve as the 'on' signal for histamine release while cyclic AMP is the 'off' signal.

Stimulation of phospholipid methylation allows Ca^{2+} to enter the cell. Cyclic AMP then inhibits methyltransferase and Ca^{2+} influx is stopped. However, once a packet of Ca^{2+} enters the cell its further actions cannot be prevented by cyclic AMP.

Rat leukemic basophils (RLB) also secrete histamine which is triggered by an IgE mediated receptor[2]. Because these cells can be cultured and modified by mitogens they serve as a useful model to study the complex biochemical events from the activation of IgE receptors to the release of histamine. Preincubation of RLB with [^{3}H]methyl-methionine followed by stimulation of IgE antigen led to a transient increase in the incorporation of [^{3}H]methyl group into phospholipids[8]. After 5 min the [^{3}H]methyl phospholipids declined. The release of histamine closely paralleled the decline in the methylated phospholipids. The relationship between phospholipid methylation and histamine release was further investigated by using varying concentrations of the methyltransferase inhibitor, 3-deaza-adenosine. Increasing concentrations of 3-deaza-adenosine resulted in a dose-dependent inhibition of the release of histamine and in the incorporation of [^{3}H]methyl groups into phospholipids.

The close temporal relationship between the antigen-stimulated release of histamine and the decline of [^{3}H]methylated phospholipids indicated that the secretion of histamine might involve further metabolism of the methylated phospholipids. One possible metabolic route would be by the hydrolytic cleavage of phosphatidylcholine by phospholipase A_2. Ca^{2+} is required to activate phospholipase A_2 and this may explain one of the functions of this cation in the release of histamine. As a measure of phospholipase A_2 activity, phosphatidylcholine was prelabelled with [^{14}C]arachidonic acid[8]. This fatty acid is preferentially incorporated into phosphatidylcholine via the methylation pathway[9]. Arachidonic acid also gives rise to many physiologically-active metabolites such as prostaglandins and leukotrienes. The addition of an IgE antigen to RLB caused a marked release of [^{14}C]arachidonic acid and its metabolites into the media. This release paralleled the secretion of histamine. Further evidence that arachidonic acid arises from phosphatidylcholine synthesized mainly via the methylation pathway was obtained by the use of methyltransferase inhibitors. The addition of 3-DZA to RLB blocked the receptor mediated release of arachidonic acid. The methyltransferase inhibitor also markedly reduced the influx of Ca^{2+}. 3-DZA blocked Ca^{2+} influx, arachidonic acid release and histamine secretion at concentrations that inhibited phospholipid methylation but not protein or nucleic acid methylation.

The liberation of arachidonic acid arising from phosphatidylcholine by IgE antigens suggested that activation of phospholipase A_2 may play an important role in the release of histamine. Inhibition of phospholipase A_2 by mepacrine or α-parabromoacetophenone blocked the release of histamine as well as arachidonic acid[10]. Arachidonic acid released by phospholipase A_2 after stimulation of RBL was mainly metabolized to prostaglandin D_2. Inhibition of the metabolism of arachidonic acid via the cyclo-oxygenase pathway with indometacin did not prevent the release of histamine, suggesting that prostaglandins are not involved in histamine release from RBL. This leaves the possibility that leukotrienes, metabolites of arachidonic acid via the lipoxygenase pathway, and/or lysolecithin, metabolites of phospholipase A_2, are components in the release of histamine.

Numerous variants of RBL cells can be obtained by the use of mutagens. Sublines of RBL mutants that did not release histamine and failed to show an influx of Ca^{2+} by IgE antigens isolated by the use of antibiotics were cloned and examined for phospholipid methyltransferase activity[11]. Among the various mutants examined, two were found to be defective in phospholipid methyltransferases, one had a low specific activity for phospholipid methyltransferase I and the other had a reduced activity of phospholipid methyltransferase II. Fusion of the two defective mutants restored both enzyme activities and the influx of Ca^{2+} and histamine secretion upon IgE receptor stimulation. These results gave further support for the importance of phospholipid methylation in the release of histamine from cells.

All of these observations suggest that in rat mast cells the IgE receptor, methyltransferase enzymes, adenylate cyclase, Ca^{2+} ion channel, phospholipase A_2 and phosphatidylcholine rich in arachidonic acid are closely clustered in the membrane (Fig. 1). When IgE receptors on the surface of mast cells or RLB are bridged by IgE specific antigens or antibodies to the receptor a cascade of events is triggered. Methyltransferases are stimulated and as has been found in erythrocytes, synaptosomes and liver endoplasmic reticulum, the phospholipids are probably translocated from the cytoplasmic to the outer surface of the membrane as they are methylated. This then would bring phosphatidylcholine in juxtaposition to phospholipase A_2 on the outer surface of the membrane (Fig. 1). The increased methylation also leads to the influx of Ca^{2+} possibly by local changes in fluidity of the membrane. The increased intracellular Ca^{2+} activates phospholipase A_2 which then hydrolyzes phosphatidylcholine rich in arachidonic acid. The metabolic products of phospholipase, lysolecithin and arachidonic acid by a still unknown mechanism causes a release of histamine. IgE receptors activate adenylate cyclase and the synthesis of cyclic AMP shortly after phospholipid methylation is stimulated. Cyclic AMP then inhibits phospholipid methylation which then shuts off further influx of Ca^{2+} necessary for the release of histamine.

Reading list

1 Goth, A. and Johnson, A. R. (1975) *Life Sci.* 16, 1201–1213
2 Ishizaka, K. and Ishizaka, T. (1969) *J. Immunol.* 103, 588–595
3 Hirata, F. and Axelrod, J. (1980) *Science* 209, 1082–1090
4 Nakajima, M., Tamura, E., Irimura, T., Toyoshima, S., Hirano, H. and Osawa, T. (1981) *J. Biochem.* 89, 665–676
5 Ishizaka, T., Hirata, F., Ishizaka, K. and Axelrod, J. (1980) *Proc. Natl Acad. Sci. U.S.A.* 77, 1903–1906
6 Cantoni, G. L., Richards, H. H. and Chiang, P. K. (1979) in *Transmethylation* (Usdin, E., Borchardt, R. T. and Creveling, C. R., eds), Vol. 5, pp. 155–164, Elsevier/North-Holland Inc., New York
7 Ishizaka, T., Hirata, F., Sterk, A. R., Ishizaka, K. and Axelrod, J. (1981) *Proc. Natl Acad. Sci. U.S.A.* 78, 6812–6816
8 Crews, F. T., Hirata, F., Axelrod, J. and Siraganian, R. P. (1980) *Biochem. Biophys. Res. Commun.* 93, 42–49
9 Crews, F. T., Morita, Y., McGivney, A., Hirata, F., Siraganian, R. P. and Axelrod, J. (1981) *Arch. Biochem. Biophys.* 212, 561–571
10 McGivney, A., Morita, Y., Crews, F. T., Hirata, F., Axelrod, J. and Siraganian, R. P. (1981) *Arch. Biochem. Biophys.* 212, 572–580
11 McGivney, A., Crews, F. T., Hirata, F., Axelrod, J. and Siraganian, R. P. (1981) *Proc. Natl Acad. Sci. U.S.A.* 78, 6176–6180
12 Hirata, F., del Carmine, R., Nelson, C. A., Axelrod, J., Schiffmann, E., Warabi, A., De Blas, A. L., Nirenberg, M., Manganiello, V., Vaughan, M., Kumagai, S., Green, I., Decker, J. L. and Steinberg, A. D. (1981) *Proc. Natl Acad. Sci. U.S.A.* 78, 3190–3194

Putatively intracellular adrenoceptors contribute to the positive inotropic effect of noradrenaline

F. Ebner

Institut für Pharmakologie und Toxikologie der Technischen Universität München, Biedersteinerstrasse 29, D-8000 München 40, F.R.G.

In the following it will be shown how a simple semiquantitative analysis of concentration–effect curves permits us to postulate that part of the positive inotropic effect of noradrenaline in guinea-pig papillary muscle is mediated by intracellularly located adrenoceptors that do not belong to the β-type.

Drug–receptor theory predicts that, if we deal with freely accessible receptors, a competitive antagonist should cause a strictly parallel shift of concentration–effect curves to higher concentrations of the agonist. The degree of this shift depends on the affinity of the antagonist to the receptor and its concentration. In guinea-pig papillary muscle, the positive inotropic effects (ΔF_c) obtained with isoprenaline in the absence and presence of propranolol (a competitive antagonist at β-adrenoceptors) fulfil these expectations (Fig. 1A). The additional presence of phentolamine was without any influence.

Drug–receptor theory further predicts

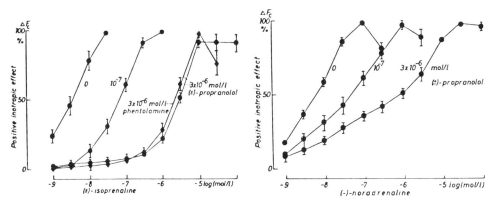

Fig. 1. (A) The isoprenaline–propranolol antagonism. (B) the noradrenaline–propranolol antagonism. Ordinates: positive inotropic effect (ΔF_c) in percent of maximal catecholamine effect. Abscissa: logarithm of molar concentration of the catecholamine. 1 Hz stimulation frequency, 6-Hydroxydopamine pretreatment. (From Ref. 2.)

that, if two agonists act on the same type of receptor, identical concentrations of an antagonist will produce the same reduction of apparent potency of both agonists. Yet, active sites of loss may interfere with the concentration of the catecholamine in the extracellular space. These processes can grossly distort the competitive antagonism and thus falsify the comparison of effects of different catecholamines[3,7], especially if the catecholamines have different affinities to these sites of loss. In guinea-pig myocardium neuronal uptake is highly effective. This becomes evident after chemical sympathectomy with 6-hydroxydopamine. This procedure did not appreciably affect the sensitivity of the muscle to isoprenaline (known to be a very poor substrate of neuronal uptake), but caused a more than 100-fold increase in the sensitivity to noradrenaline[2], just as a high concentration (2×10^{-5} mol l^{-1}) of cocaine did[3]. (Note: the experiments of Fig. 1A were carried out after pretreatment of the animals with 6-hydroxydopamine.) In spite of chemical sympathectomy and in spite of overwhelming evidence that noradrenaline and isoprenaline act upon the same cardiac β-adrenoceptors, the results appearing in Fig. 1B (noradrenaline – propranolol antagonism) are very different from those of Fig. 1A (isoprenaline – propranolol antagonism). While the shift of both catecholamine effects by propranolol is quite similar at the high levels of effect, there is a pronounced (and unexpected) decrease in the slope of the curve with noradrenaline. Indeed we are justified in speaking of a 'propranolol-resistant' effect of noradrenaline at the levels of low effect. This peculiar type of antagonism was not restricted to pretreatment with 6-hydroxydopamine. It was similar when neuronal uptake was eliminated by cocaine[3]. Clearly these experiments with noradrenaline are inconsistent with the concept of a simple competitive antagonism.

Since we excluded only one site of loss (neuronal uptake) by pretreatment with 6-hydroxydopamine or by cocaine, we must also consider the possible involvement of extraneuronal uptake. If it were an important second site of loss in this preparation, one would expect an inhibitor of extraneuronal uptake, hydrocortisone, to cause supersensitivity to noradrenaline. However, hydrocortisone not only failed to cause supersensitivity but actually reduced the effect of noradrenaline in such a way that the 'propranolol-resistant' component disappeared (see Fig. 2, hatched area). As a consequence, the picture of a 'simple competitive antagonism' (noradrenaline – propranolol) was unmasked, if the experiments were carried out in the presence of hydrocortisone (compare triangles of Fig. 2 with the corresponding curves of Fig. 1A).

Interestingly, phentolamine (Fig. 3) and phenoxybenzamine had the same effect as hydrocortisone. Neither altered the noradrenaline control appreciably and both changed the antagonism of propranolol into a parallel one by interfering with the 'propranolol-resistant' component of the noradrenaline effect. As there had been no such effect of isoprenaline, there was also no inhibitory effect of phentolamine (see Fig. 1A).

These results are compatible with the view that, (a) both catecholamines interact with freely accessible β-adrenoceptors for which they compete with propranolol and, (b) noradrenaline, but not isoprenaline, exerts a hydrocortisone-sensitive effect on a second set of adrenoceptors that are resistant to propranolol.

Since hydrocortisone lacks any ability to block β-adrenoceptors[5], while it is known to inhibit extraneuronal uptake, the effects of hydrocortisone described here may well reflect its ability to block extraneuronal uptake. But if extraneuronal uptake is ineffective as a site of loss from the extracellular space, its blockade cannot induce supersensitivity of those effects which are mediated by the adrenoceptors of the cellular surface. Actually, it was shown that in contrast to other species and tissues, extraneuronal uptake is poorly developed in guinea-pig myocardium[1,2]. Rates of hydrocortisone-sensitive O-methylation were far lower in guinea-pig papillary muscle than in any other tissue studied thus far[2]. In view of these observations it is tempting to propose that, while blockade of uptake with hydrocortisone was insufficient to induce supersensitivity, it did unmask an effector site of noradrenaline which was located beyond extraneuronal uptake. It is suggested that in guinea-pig myocardium, extraneuronal uptake does not function as a 'site of loss' for the extracellular space, rather, it represents the 'site of gain' which mediates the access of the catecholamine to an intracellular space.

This putatively intracellular adrenoceptor could be of the β-type, provided isoprenaline was metabolized more actively than noradrenaline, thereby preventing an accumulation in the interior of the muscle cell. However, inhibition of metabolism (catechol-O-methyl-transferase and monoamine oxidase) altered neither the noradrenaline nor the isoprenaline effects[2]. This lack of effect was corroborated by the low rates of O-methylation[2]. Likewise one might propose that at intracellular β-adrenoceptors a highly permeable, i.e. highly lipophilic, antagonist (propranolol) would be more potent than the hydrophilic practolol (octanol/water partition coefficients at pH = 7: propranolol = 5.39, practolol = 0.009; data from Ref. 6). Yet, the experiment showed no difference between the antagonists. Thus, it appears that this putatively intracellular adrenoceptor is not of the β-type. Beyond this statement, a definitive classification is not yet possible. The results obtained with phentolamine and phenoxybenzamine do not prove the existence of α-adrenoceptors, since both receptor antagonists not only inhibit α-adrenoceptors but also extraneuronal uptake[4]. Consequently, the existence of α-adrenoceptors can no longer be inferred from the inhibitory activity of phentolamine or phenoxybenzamine, if extraneuronal uptake may be involved as a pathway leading to an intracellular effector site. For a differentiation one would need an antagonist at

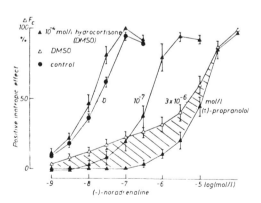

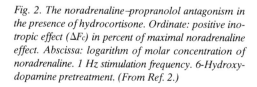

Fig. 2. The noradrenaline–propranolol antagonism in the presence of hydrocortisone. Ordinate: positive inotropic effect (ΔF_c) in percent of maximal noradrenaline effect. Abscissa: logarithm of molar concentration of noradrenaline. 1 Hz stimulation frequency. 6-Hydroxydopamine pretreatment. (From Ref. 2.)

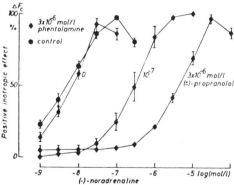

Fig. 3. The noradrenaline–propranolol antagonism in the presence of phentolamine. Ordinate: positive inotropic effect (ΔF_c) in percent of maximal noradrenaline effect. Abscissa: logarithm of molar concentration of noradrenaline. 1 Hz stimulation frequency. 6-Hydroxydopamine pretreatment. (From Ref. 2.)

α-adrenoceptors which is lipophilic enough to enter the cell but fails to affect extraneuronal uptake. Unfortunately, such an agent is not available at present. Only the difference of the effect of noradrenaline from that of isoprenaline supports an involvement of α-adrenoceptors.

In conclusion, experiments have presented evidence in favour of a postsynaptic difference of action of noradrenaline and isoprenaline in guinea-pig papillary muscle. They suggest an exclusive activation of intracellular adrenoceptors by noradrenaline. Though different from β-adrenoceptors, they cannot yet be classified definitely as α-adrenoceptors.

Reading list

1 Bönisch, H. and Trendelenburg, U. (1974) *Naunyn-Schmiedebergs Arch. Pharmakol.* 283, 191–218
2 Ebner, F. (1981) *Naunyn-Schmiedebergs Arch. Pharmakol.* 316, 8–18
3 Ebner, F. (1981) *Naunyn-Schmiedebergs Arch. Pharmakol.* 316, 96–107
4 Eisenfeld, A. J., Axelrod, J. and Krakoff, L. (1967) *J. Pharmacol. Exp. Ther.* 156, 107–113
5 Graefe, K.-H. and Trendelenburg, U. (1974) *Naunyn-Schmiedebergs Arch. Pharmakol.* 286, 1–48
6 Hellenbrecht, D., Lemmer, B., Wiethold, G. and Grobecker, H. (1973) *Naunyn-Schmiedebergs Arch. Pharmakol.* 277, 211–226
7 Langer, S. Z. and Trendelenburg, U. (1969) *J. Pharmacol. Exp. Ther.* 167, 117–142

Index

Acetylcholine receptors 2, 115, 119, 125
AC⁻S49 lymphoma cells 15
ACTH 14
Adenosine deaminase 144
Adenosine receptors
   and cAMP levels 140–141
      methylxanthines 142
      P site receptors 142–147
      R site receptors 142–147
      rat neurons, effect on 108
Adenosine triphosphate 140
Adenylate cyclase
   and cAMP synthesis 29, 68
      the C unit 15, 16, 22
      the functional units 14–15
      the G/F regulatory protein 34, 35
      the GTP analogs 17, 18, 21, 34
      GTP, receptor dependence 30, 68
      guanyl nucleotides 23
      the N unit 15–17, 22
α-Adrenoceptors
   and Ca^{2+} 70–74
      cAMP 68, 74
      general properties of 66
      GTP analogs 67, 68
      guanyl nucleotides 67
β-Adrenoceptors
   and adenylate cyclase 32–38, 48–53
      affinity chromatography 34, 35
      cAMP production 14, 25, 33
      anti-receptor antibodies 36–38
      catecholamine responsive cells 49, 52
      isoproterenol 33, 52
      noradrenergic neuronal activity 48
ADTN 78
Alprenolol 45
AMP, cyclic 8, 29, 49, 77, 84, 87, 140, 148, 149, 169, 171
   and ACh 118
      DA receptors 77
      'non-cyclase' hormones 8
      insulin 149
      theophylline 169
Anti-alprenolol 38
Antibodies, receptor 9, 40
Apomorphine 79, 80, 81, 83, 85, 99
ATP 29, 30, 140, 149, 150, 165
Auto-antibodies 42

Barbiturates 111
Basic-somatomedin 4, 9
Benzamides 77
Benzodiazepines 105
Burimamide 134
Butyrophenones 77, 78, 81, 82, 84, 85, 89

Ca^{2+} 55, 66, 69, 70–73, 162–166, 168, 171
cAMP 61–65, 69, 73, 74, 162
   See also AMP, cyclic
Carbachol 4
cGMP 61–65
Chloroquine 26
Cholera toxin 16, 17, 64
Cimetidine 134–136
Clonidine 66–74
Coated pits 10, 52
Colchicine 30
Concanavalin A 150

Dansylcadavarin 52
Desensitization 29
Diazepam 4–5
Disuccinimidyl suberate 3
Dopamine
   and auto-receptors 93
      behavioural regulation in mammals 95
      binding sites in mammalian brain 94
      classification of its receptors 76–85, 87, 88, 93–97
      receptor cascade 76
      the SIF cell 58

EGF-URO 2–5, 8–10, 45
Enkephalin 23
Epinephrine 14, 70, 71, 74
Estradiol 123
Etintidine 139
Etomidate 112

Fab fragments 8, 44
Flupenthixol 78, 83, 89
Flurazepam 108

GABA 4, 5, 91, 105, 106, 111–114
GDP 16, 20
Glucagon 10, 14, 21, 34

Glycogen synthase 148
Gonadotropin receptors 15
Gramicidin 121
GTP 7, 16, 17, 18–23, 29, 36, 42, 50, 120, 146
Guanosine 108
Guanylate cyclase 62
Guanyl nucleotides 22, 23, 67, 68

Hagfish 155
Haloperidol 82, 89, 101
Histamine
  and activation of adenylate cyclase 14
    activation of phospholipase A2 170
    antagonists 134
    its release 167
    classification of histamine receptors 134
    ranitidine, reaction to 136–138
Hydrocortisone 173
Hydroxymethylglutaryl CoA reductase 148
Hypercholesterolemia 12
Hypoxanthine 107, 108

Immunological techniques 40
Insulin
  and affinity-labeling 155, **156**
    internalisation of receptor complex 150
    receptor structure 3, 156–161
    phosphorylation 148–153
Inosine 107, 108
Interferon 3, 9
Isoprenaline 30, 174
Isoproterenol 51

Ligand recognition 3
Low density lipoprotein 12

α-Methylnorepinephrine 67, 68
Methylxanthines 140, 142, 146
Mitochondria 70
Morphine 23, 45
Muscarinic receptor 4, 115–118, 119–124

Nerve growth factor 9
Nicotinamide 107–109
Nitroglycerine 64
Noradrenaline 57, 172–175
Norepinephrine synthesis 48, 49

Oligomeric receptors 1–6, 10–12
Oligosaccharide 2

Papaverine 96
Parkinson's disease 94, 98, 99

Pentobarbitone 112
Phenethylamine 104
Phenothiazines 77, 84
Phentolamine 26, 172
Phosphatidylcholine 167
Phosphatidylethanolamine 113
Phosphatidylinositol 66, 71, 72, 74, 118, 162–166
Phosphodiesterase 30, 64
Phospholipase A2 170
Phosphorylation 11, 56
  See also Insulin
Picrotoxinin 112
Piribedil 81, 96
Platelet membranes 23
3 PPP 98–104
Prazosin 66–74
Progesterone 123
Prolactin 5, 84
Propranolol 45, 62
Prostaglandin E$_1$ 68
Protein I 57
Protein kinase 62–65
Protein oligomers 1
Pseudohypoparathyroidism 12
Purine metabolism 140
Purinergic receptors 140
Pyruvate dehydrogenase 148, 149, 151

Ranitidine 136–139
  See also Histamine
Receptors
  Acetylcholine 1, 3, 41, 43, 115, 119, 125
  Adenosine 55, 140–147
  α-adrenoceptors 66–74
  β-adrenoceptors 7, 12, 15–23, 25–31, 32–38, 45, 48–52, 57, 61, 172–175
  Barbiturate 111–114
  Benzodiazepine 105–110
  Dopamine 55, 76–85, 87–91, 93–97, 98–104
  Epidermal Growth Factor 1, 8
  GABA 4, 106, 111–114
  Glucagon 7
  Histamine 134
  Immunoglobulin E 167–172
  Insulin 2, 8, 42, 148–161
  Muscarinic 41, 115–124
  Nerve Growth Factor 3
  Nicotinic 41, 115, 125–132
  Opiate 23
  Parathyroid hormone 12
  Serotonin 55
  Thyroid stimulating hormone 42
Reductase kinase 148

S49 lymphoma cells 37
Schizophrenia 98

Secretin   34
Serotonin   59
SIF cell   58
Sodium butyrate   5
Solubilised plasma membranes   40
Spiroperidol   89
Sulpiride   89
Synaptic transmission   54

Tetrodotoxin   121
Theophylline   58, 142, 146, 169
Thrombin   164

Thromboxane A_2 107, 109
Tiotidine   138
Torpedo fish   3, 32, 125

Ulcer therapy   134

Valinomycin   121
Vasodilation   77, 80, 134
Vasointestinal peptide   14
Veratridine   121

Yohimbine   66–74